Nutritional Compass

A Natural Guide to Today's Food Choices

*Jaime Camirand, BAS, R.H.N. and
Dr. Elvis Ali, ND*

ACKNOWLEDGMENTS

I would like to express my sincere gratitude to those who have contributed support, inspiration, assistance and motivation:

My family and friends for all of their love, understanding and encouragement: Rafath, my parents, Carmen and Michael, and my brother, Alex, as well my grandparents from whom I have continued to learn long after they have gone.

Friends, colleagues and educators at the University of Guelph, Canadian School of Natural Nutrition; Lyn-Dys Health Food and Nature's Signature for their expertise, insight and enlightenment.

Dr. Elvis Ali and publisher/editor Sherree Felstead, who have made essential contributions in helping knowledge and ideas come to life.

- Jaime Camirand

It is a pleasure to acknowledge with thanks:

My entire family in Canada and Trinidad and Tobago who have continued to support, and motivate me to educate others about naturopathic medicine. My parents, Hakim, Hazrah, my sisters, Alima, Homaida, Homeeda, Fazida, my children, Hassan, Azeeda, Kareem; nephews, nieces and precious grandchildren, Gursimran, Meheirveer and Shairveer for their encouragement and belief in holistic medicine.

Colleagues in the healthcare profession, specifically Dr. Leo Roy and Albert E. D'Souza B.Sc.

My students and staff at CCNM, BINM, CCHH, OAND, CAND and clinics, BTNL, AA Comfort Health Centers and Mississauga clinic.

The companies for their assistance in educating the public about preventative medicine: Biorrific, Ecoideas, Canadian Bio, Sangsters, Fion Beauty Supplies Canada, Alpha Science Laboratories – A division of Omega Alpha Pharmaceuticals Inc.

My dear friends, Bonita, Pat, Roy, Cindy and Darryl, Janak, Joan, Ash and Harry, Saira and Moe Sheikh of Etobicoke Motors, along with many others too numerous to list.

Graphic designer Lillian who designed the book cover, and of course, Sherree my editor and publisher.

- Dr. Elvis Ali

CONTENTS

"Fascinating and informative, much of which I tried to practice back in the 70s, but with having to prepare for someone else who eats differently, it became difficult to continue. This book is concise and well structured, and easy to read."- Gloria Mullett (Age 81)

FOREWORD

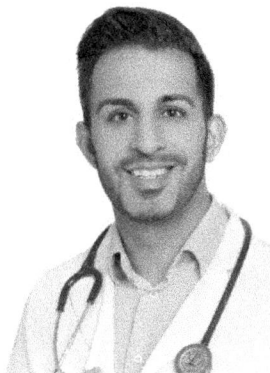

Creating a bridge between traditional western medicine and natural, preventative medicine has always been my primary focus and passion. As an MD, health and fitness coach, and studying naturopathic medicine, my philosophy is to treat the *whole* person by providing the right balance of medical diagnosis with healthy lifestyle choices that encourages optimal health and wellbeing. Empowering patients to be more proactive in making sound, healthful choices, in my view, creates a far lesser burden of disease to enjoy a more vibrant life into old age.

I was delighted when I found out that one of my most inspiring mentors, Dr. Elvis Ali is co-authoring with one of his colleagues, nutritionist, Jaime Camirand, a nutritional guide for healthy eating. Healthy eating is one of the most important aspects of preventative medicine. Hippocrates, considered the father of medicine, said: "Let food be thy medicine and medicine be thy food." During his time, around 460 BC, food provided the most nutrients for the body's needs, without the complex environmental conditions we face today. Furthermore, it is worth noting that healthy eating strengthens and supports the body's healing when having to take prescribed pharmaceuticals.

Nutritional Compass is very informative, and lifts the veil of confusion surrounding today's foods. It covers choosing your foods at the grocery store to cooking them at home. It breaks down the science of nutrition into simple, and useful terms so you know how specific foods work for your body in order to achieve your most favorable health. This book covers not only the macronutrients (carbohydrates, protein fats), and micro nutrients, but also goes further to explain the science of the popular superfoods, such as Maca and **Spirulina,** and tells you how to incorporate them into your diet.

The advice on nutrition and the perspective of a healthy lifestyle presented by both Dr. Elvis and Jaime is distinct from all other experts in the field. *Nutritional Compass* does an excellent job in teaching the everyday individual how to develop a healthy and nutritious lifestyle that works for them.

Sandip Oppal, MD
Health and Fitness Coach,
ND (Candidate)

NATURE
Is so smart, it put medicine inside the food.

The foundation of optimal health and healing is sound mind-body-soul. From modern traditional crisis intervention medicine practiced today, to the ancient healing systems of China, India, Indigenous peoples and other societies worldwide, the 21st century is the gateway to a new exciting health, and healing reality - one which offers the opportunity for a longer and better quality of life, at all stages of life. Natural, organic foods will be a crucial aspect of helping to achieve and maintain the most favourable health and wellness.

When disease, illness or injury strikes, the 20th century's crisis intervention allopathic medical model deals mainly with the symptoms, using diagnostic tools, prescription drugs and surgical techniques based on a dispassionate scientific perception of medicine. If one is having a heart attack, has a hernia or physical trauma, requiring immediate attention, modern allopathic medicine must be the first option. However, in terms of prevention and long-term quality of life, this system pays little attention to the powerful role of the mind, body and soul, and healthy eating, preferring to focus on the symptoms, not the underlying cause that must be corrected.

Chinese, Indian, Anthroposophical and other healing models focus on using the most powerful healing source: your own body's wisdom to heal itself, and help you attain and maintain a state of optimal wellbeing. We believe in preventive medicine that begins with proper nutrition, along with holistic medicine, which is a more integrated approach that values the mind, body and soul balance.

The new model of health and healing uses the best of *all* the models, with a focus on prevention and healing by using less intrusive interventions, and guiding the body in the direction best suited to provoke the required healing response needed at that time. Symptoms are seen as signs of deeper underlying problems that have to be resolved or the symptom might return and negatively impact the quality of one's life. The body, unfortunately, will age more rapidly than normal.

Nutritional Compass gives you a blend of thoughts that are directed to consuming quality foods and diet recommendations to enhance what our hectic and stressful lifestyles have become. It adjusts for the unnatural foods we eat, environments we live in and medical approaches we typically use by giving you gentle, natural aids to help you live longer and enhance your body's natural abilities to heal.

INTRODUCTION

At times, it can be easy to forget how central food is to life. Food is survival, fuel, nourishment and medicine. Harnessing energy from the earth and sun, it provides the basic necessities for life, and is likely the most crucial determinant of overall health and wellbeing. Food is also fun, celebration art and culture. It is a reflection of our physical, social and economic environments.

In a world where so many people don't have enough to survive, some of us are extremely fortunate to have access to a virtually limitless food supply. However, this overwhelming number of food choices has become an issue of its own, as many of these choices show less and less resemblance to real food. Some societies have now found themselves in a state of excess, filled with obesity rather than famine. Yet, in the midst of this enormous surplus, nutritional deficiencies and chronic diseases continue to increase. Many people become so busy working to afford their survival that they neglect to consider the food that defines it. However, for those who are lucky enough to have choices regarding their health, optimal wellbeing can be achieved with the help of accurate nutritional knowledge and awareness.

When compared to the food of our ancestors, the modern food industry is almost unrecognizable. The past few decades have seen some massive increases in population, and consequently in food production. This shift has brought about a whole new era of fast, cheap and preserved foods made to travel long distances and feed more people for less money. Today, the food industry is a crowded and convoluted market worth trillions of dollars, which is mostly owned by a small handful of powerful corporations. In the interest of increasing profits, much of the food supply is grown and produced using the cheapest methods and ingredients that will fit within the boundaries of current food protection laws. With minimal regard for human or environmental health, many methods and additives are used on our food before they can be adequately studied, and several are subsequently banned in several countries.

While this view of the food industry may look bleak, there is another more encouraging movement that seems to be growing by the minute: a return to natural, whole, pure, nourishment from the earth. Consumer awareness and demand is a powerful force, proven by the skyrocketing availability of whole, additive-free and organic food options. This is a huge triumph for human health, and is changing the face of the food industry for the better.

However, with this rising interest in wholesome eating, comes more and more information about the best ways to execute it. Nutritional research is constantly overturning new rocks and presenting new theories, and has provided a large collection of very useful, yet sometimes contradictory or incomplete information regarding human nutrition. Combined with varying personal opinions and philosophical ideas about nutrition, the scientific atmosphere has become disorienting. It seems that everywhere you look, there is a new announcement about the "perfect" way to eat, a new list of foods to avoid, or a new bandwagon dedicated to another restrictive diet trend. This increased awareness and large volume of information available about health, food and nutrition is a wonderful thing. The challenge is sifting through this information to find simple, accurate comprehension and using it in a way that is supportive to health.

A Shift in Perspective

Food's fundamental purpose is to fuel and nourish, and to understand and respect it as such is crucial to maintaining a healthy, rewarding relationship with it. Yes, we all have a relationship with food. It's up to us whether that relationship is destructive and dysfunctional, or enjoyable and rewarding. This difference begins with attitude.

There is no doubt that maintaining a perfect diet in a modern, fast-paced society is difficult. Eating well is a challenge. It takes time, effort, dedication and patience. But the toughest challenge is a matter of mentality. Most people find themselves in this dilemma at one time or another –a mission to eat "healthier" for the purpose of weight loss, overall health or maybe just because that's what we're all expected to do as responsible adults. However, this mission becomes nearly impossible when it is viewed as a form of deprivation or restriction.

Any physical action, if accompanied by a negative attitude, will not be effective and sustainable. This means that eating nutritious foods with resistance and disgust may not be very healthy in the long run. In fact, human cells are shown to change and react in response to positive and negative thinking. Stress and negativity take a significant toll on overall health, including the way we digest foods. On a psychological level, associating healthy living with feelings of resentment will make it a lot less appealing and much harder to stick with.

Food choices can be seen as a very direct representation of a person's intentions for his or her own life. Choosing whole, "live" foods over refined, preserved, "lifeless" foods is very much the same as choosing to nourish and support your body rather than to place a burden on it. As a result, food choices become much more than just eating. They are an opportunity to express love and gratitude for our bodies, our minds, our planet, and the food that comes from it. Maintaining a healthy diet and lifestyle is much more achievable when it comes naturally. This might mean changing your outlook on health, and viewing food as nourishment and fuel rather than indulgence or habit. A genuine appreciation for your food and your health will create an automatic shift in the way you think about eating, resulting in essentially effortless diet and lifestyle changes.

Living a truly healthy life depends on respect for oneself along with an understanding of the world around us and what it offers. What this book offers is a clear and positive perspective – delivering the nutritional knowledge needed to navigate the complicated terrain of the modern food industry, and simplifying your journey toward natural wellness.

PART I

Understanding the Nature of Today's Foods

"This magical, marvelous food on our plate, this sustenance we absorb, has a story to tell. It has a journey. It leaves a footprint. It leaves a legacy. To eat with reckless abandon, without conscience, without knowledge, folks, this isn't normal." – Joel Salatin, farmer and author of *Folks, This Ain't Normal*;*You Can Farm*

1

The Evolution of Nourishment

The development of what has come to be known as "food" has a very long and elaborate history.

The earth, and the organisms that live upon it, have interacted and grown with one another for millions of years. The sun happened to be in the perfect position to provide just enough heat and energy to support life. Plants have evolved to harness this energy – not only to grow and survive, but also to create energy and give life to other organisms. Human beings evolved alongside these plants for a very long time, with capabilities to digest and assimilate them. Just as plants recycle carbon dioxide and produce life-giving oxygen, they provide an array of **different nutrients including vitamins, minerals, amino acids, antioxidants and other phytochemicals in specific combinations and ratios.**

It is no coincidence that the nutrients found in plants are the same ones that humans and other animals require for survival and wellbeing. In most cases, these nutrients are even found in perfect quantities within the ideal ecosystems and environments. For example, today's humans have evolved to require Vitamin C from foods, rather than producing it themselves as almost all other animals do. It turns out that this nutrient can be obtained from several different fruits and vegetables, including watery, cooling fruits, such as pineapple, papaya, kiwi and citrus fruits, which grow in hot, humid climates. Many fruits of this kind also contain edible seeds that have historically been consumed by humans and passed through the digestive tract unharmed as a form of seed dispersal, benefitting the survival of both animals and plants.

Of course, each plant has evolved differently and they all have varying interactions with human health. History and evolution are not necessarily the only considerations when it comes to nutrition, but they certainly have a significant place in the story. The symbiotic relationships between humans, plants, animals, bacteria and virtually every other substance on earth are extremely complex and extraordinary in more ways than we can even imagine. Nothing compares to what the earth can offer us, and respecting and understanding that fact is crucial to human health and the health of the planet.

Food Modification: Where Did We Go Wrong?

A truly "whole" food is a complete, unaltered product of the earth that has evolved with all of its original constituents and natural energy to provide nourishment for another entity. However, even whole foods are often changed in some way before consumption. As human beings have evolved, so has the way that they consume food from the earth. Many foods are only edible with some effort, including peeling, cutting or heating. Some foods actually exhibit increased bioavailability of certain nutrients when altered; for example, cooking, soaking or sprouting will unlock certain nutrients while removing anti-nutrients that prevent absorption. Similarly, other important health-promoting components, such as the allicin found in garlic, are only released when the plant is crushed.

Unfortunately, food modification can be a slippery slope. As technology advances and food continues to grow as an industry, food is becoming almost unrecognizable. Methods like processing, preserving, refining and extracting often remove a large portion of a food's original constituents, thus affecting the way it is digested and assimilated. A common example of this is the refining of sugar. In its natural state, sugar is often accompanied by fibre, B vitamins, amino acids and other nutrients that modulate its absorption and allow it to be utilized safely and effectively. However, refined, white sugar and similar products like high-fructose corn syrup have become increasingly dominant ingredients in many foods. In exaggerated amounts, and away from all of its original constituents, sugar can do some very serious damage. Refined sugars exclude useful nutrients that help to regulate digestion and absorption, and instead subject the human body to a very large and unregulated dose of sugar, which contributes to almost every disease imaginable, including diabetes, cardiovascular disease, cancer, mental illness and addiction.

Even whole foods may not be truly "whole" anymore. Mass production has affected not only the way food is processed, but also the way it is grown, introducing issues like mono-cropping, pesticide use, genetic modification, soil depletion, loss of variety and destruction of ecosystems. Changes in the soil and the surrounding ecosystems, let alone a plant's DNA, will ultimately affect its nutrient content, and the way that it affects human health. A plant that grows naturally in nutrient-rich soil, surrounded by a large variety of other living things, will exhibit a very different nutrient profile than one that has been grown in restrictive conditions, depleted soil and in the presence of only other identical, genetically engineered species. This discrepancy can even be demonstrated by the differences between modern crops and the crops that were grown 50 years ago. For example, 100g of fresh tomatoes in 2006 contained 30.7 percent less Vitamin A and 16.9 percent less Vitamin C than 100g of the 1963 equivalent. To make matters of nutrient depletion even worse, food is often harvested prematurely to preserve freshness, unable to develop its full nutrient profile. Then, it begins losing nutrients the moment it is picked, resulting in much lower concentrations once it has travelled across countries, continents or around the world. It's clear that our food supply is not as nourishing as it once was, even if we are making healthy, whole food choices. Buying food from small, local farms that use more natural growing practices might help to resolve this issue. In an ideal world, societies would transition back toward a healthier, more diverse and sustainable method of farming, improving both human and environmental health. With increased awareness and demand, this may be more realistic than one would think.

Whole Food: Greater than the Sum of Its Parts

Due to the prevalence of empty, processed foods, as well as steady nutrient depletion of several crops, many countries are plagued by nutritional deficiencies and related illnesses. Many people have also come to simply not have the time or motivation to eat "real" food, and instead, rely on fast, convenient or packaged foods. As a result, nutritional supplementation and fortification have been rapidly gaining popularity as a substitute for natural, whole food nutrition.

We are fortunate enough to have access to a vast and growing collection of knowledge about nutrition. Science has revealed some amazing information about nutrients and their roles in human health. Conversely, advancements in science and technology have led to an entirely different way of obtaining, and simultaneously omitting, the nutrients required for human health. Nutritional research often involves studying one chemical at a time to determine certain hypothesized effects on the body. This has led to trends of supplementation and fortification of packaged foods that are able to claim health benefits, but it doesn't provide nearly enough information to understand the interactions of naturally occurring nutrients with human health.

Thankfully, science has also helped to validate the power of whole food nutrition. It is now known that nutrients behave much differently in their natural states than they do in synthetic, amplified and isolated forms. Naturally occurring vitamins and minerals will be consumed along with an entire network of additional nutrients, phytochemicals, and other supporting substances that work together to provide optimal absorption. This network may enhance, slow or modulate absorption in ways that are often ideal for human health. Each plant has its own unique system of nutrients and other chemicals that synergistically interact and influence one another. In fact, there are so many different potential chemical components, combinations and interactions that it is likely impossible to accurately identify or replicate the nutritional action of a whole food. Altering and isolating nutrients could entirely change the way that they act within the body, presenting concerns of not only effectiveness, but safety.

There is a misconception that vitamin and mineral supplementation is always safe, as they are naturally occurring in food, and are known to be "good for us". However, in high amounts, improper forms and away from its supporting and modulating plant components, a nutrient does have the potential to do more harm than good. For example, some nutrients can become toxic in high amounts, especially those that continue to accumulate in the body rather than being excreted. Long-term supplementation of any one nutrient has the potential to create imbalances in relation to other nutrients as well. For example, some minerals, such as zinc and copper, exist in balance with one another. Consuming high concentrations of one may negatively affect levels of the other.

Calcium is another commonly supplemented mineral that requires the support of other nutrients like Vitamins D and K to complete its role in bone health. Taken in inorganic, poorly absorbed forms, and away from other modulating nutrients, calcium may have many more negative effects than positive. Calcium supplementation of this type has been shown to affect other functions such as blood pressure, glucose control and weight management, and may increase calcium deposition in the kidneys and arteries, resulting in higher risk of kidney stones and cardiovascular disease. Although there are varying scientific opinions about these risks with supplementation, there is no increased risk associated with food sources, indicating that food sources of calcium are likely safer and more effective in most circumstances. In another study comparing lycopene supplementation to consumption of tomatoes with naturally occurring lycopene, tomato consumption provided more favorable results on cardiovascular risk endpoints than lycopene supplementation alone.

In general, vitamins, minerals and other phytonutrients are likely safer and more effective when consumed within their natural sources. For this reason, the fortification of processed foods with synthetic vitamins, which wouldn't normally be present in those foods, is not an adequate method for preventing nutritional deficiencies. While supplementation can certainly be beneficial and even essential, it cannot replace food. Long-term supplement use should be approved by a practitioner who can ensure that each one is taken in appropriate forms, amounts and frequencies.

2

The Truth about Food Marketing

The food industry is one of the largest and most powerful industries in existence.

Food is a necessity, and the constant sale of food and food-like products contributes to a market that is worth trillions of dollars. There are endless products to choose from, which becomes further complicated by various trends and marketing strategies used to promote food products. It's important to be aware that many of these food marketing trends, while they often relate to "health", do not necessarily support optimal health at all. In general, it's best to avoid processed, packaged foods altogether by consuming mainly fresh, whole foods. However, if using any packaged foods, labels should be read carefully.

Below are some of the most common and misleading food marketing trends to watch out for.

Low Fat and Fat-Free

The anti-fat movement has made a substantial impact on the food industry. There has been a misconception among researchers, food marketers, and therefore, many consumers, that fat in food somehow signifies more fat stored in the body. In fact, adequate dietary fat is crucial to several aspects of health, including brain function, hormonal health, fertility, healthy hair and skin, and healthy weight management. Removing fats from foods and altering their composition can also affect the way that those foods are digested and metabolized. For example, fat-soluble Vitamins A, D, E, and K, found in various foods, require some dietary fats or oils along with them in order to be properly digested and assimilated.

24

Therefore, eating a nutrient-dense, leafy green salad with fat-free salad dressing won't allow you to effectively use all of the Vitamin K found in those greens. What's troubling is that many of the foods that are often produced in low-fat or fat-free forms have naturally *high* fat contents, including products like yogurt, cheese, milks, and of course, salad dressings. Altering foods in this way will remove many of the existing health benefits, and often create health nightmares when additives, such as synthetic fillers, artificial flavors and added sugars are used to compensate. The use of margarine is a perfect example of this phenomenon. For several years, margarine was promoted as a healthy alternative to butter, which was developing a reputation for negative effects on cardiovascular health. After more research, it was determined that saturated fats were not as harmful as once thought, and that they may in fact be supportive to overall health. Meanwhile, low-fat varieties of synthetically made margarine had been gaining popularity, being marketed as "heart-healthy", despite containing harmful, industrially produced trans fats that are known to increase the risk of cardiovascular disease. As a general rule, it is far better to choose a whole food product with a high amount of naturally occurring fats than to consume a product that has been chemically altered to remove or transform these fats.

Sugar-Free

With increased awareness of the harmful effects of sugar, including rising rates of diabetes, there are more and more products on the market that promise reduced or zero grams of sugar. While it is clear that excessive and refined sugars are indeed detrimental to health, one should be cautious when consuming processed foods that claim to be "sugar-free" or have "no added sugar". Removing excess sugar is an excellent choice, but this sugar is often replaced with synthetic, "sugar-free", zero-calorie sweeteners. These are often much sweeter than sugar itself, and result in a whole other list of health issues. Popular artificial sweeteners such as aspartame have been linked to varying levels of neurotoxic effects, including headaches, seizures and cell death, as well as increased risk of certain cancers. Most people now know to avoid sweeteners like aspartame, but there are several other common sweeteners that hide behind less identifiable names and guises. In most cases, it's best to avoid sweetened products altogether. For those with diabetes, artificial sweeteners should not be relied upon as a safe alternative to sugar. Sugar digestion begins in the mouth, and when a sweetener that is up to 200 times sweeter than sugar is consumed, sugar digestion and blood sugar balance are still ultimately affected. Considering this fact, along with the evidence regarding harmful effects of artificial sweeteners, those with diabetic conditions are encouraged to avoid both refined sugars and artificial sweeteners.

It's important to note that even natural sweeteners can be detrimental when consumed in excess. While some of these ingredients may be much less harmful than artificial sweeteners and refined sugar, they are still contributing to a heavily over-sweetened food market. The food industry's reliance on sugar is extremely damaging to public health, but replacing this obsession with other forms is hardly solving the problem at hand. In order to reduce dependence on sugar and maintain optimal blood sugar levels, it's crucial to avoid excess, added sugars or sweeteners, and re-train the taste buds to recognize and appreciate real food – without the need for sweeter and sweeter tastes. This reduction is important for addressing both psychological and physiological aspects of sugar addiction.

Low Calorie or Diet

Over the past few decades, there has been a growing demand in developed countries for products that promote weight loss. The food industry has certainly capitalized on this demand, and as a result, grocery store shelves are covered with words like, "low calorie", "thin", "slim", "diet" and "skinny". However, the implication that a product has a reduced amount of calories per serving does not necessarily mean that it is beneficial for health or for weight loss. As discussed above, many ingredients that are used in reduced sugar and reduced calorie products may be "zero-calorie", but introduce several other health issues. It's also important to note that often, a lower number of calories per serving are simply due to a reduction in serving size, so that ultimately the consumer is just paying more for less. When it comes to any pre-made or packaged foods, the nutritional information that includes calories, sugars and fats is based on a certain serving size, which may be much smaller than the average person would actually consume. Small servings of processed foods that contain harmful fats, refined sugars or artificial sweeteners are typically harmful to weight loss goals and health in general, resulting in further digestive and nervous system imbalances, and even more intense cravings than before.

Natural

Variations of the word "natural" are often used on food labels to imply that the product is in its natural state, and is therefore, somehow healthier or nutritionally superior. In general, any food package that emphasizes the word "natural" on it should be greeted with skepticism. Keep in mind that most foods that are contained in a package are likely not fresh or truly natural, as they have usually been altered or preserved in some way. However, it turns out that the definition of the word "natural" in the context of food labeling is more complicated than one would think.

According to the Canadian Food Inspection Agency (CFIA), a food that is represented as natural is expected to fulfill the following criteria:

- Not to contain, or to ever have contained, an added vitamin, mineral nutrient, artificial flavoring agent or food additive.

- Not to have any constituent or fraction thereof removed or significantly changed, except the removal of water. For example: the removal of caffeine.

- Not to have been submitted to processes that has significantly altered their original physical, chemical or biological state (i.e. maximum processes). - CFIA 2016

The CFIA also notes several exceptions and additions to these rules. For instance, there are two annexes describing minimum and maximum processes that affect the natural character of food. "Maximum" processes disqualify foods from being represented as natural, while "minimum" processes do not affect labeling laws. This is to say that a certain list of processes, including aging, emulsifying, fumigation and even "treatments with toxic gases (with no chemical change)" may take place without endangering the product's right to be labeled as natural. Also, any additives that are "derived from natural sources" may be considered natural. Therefore, that product may claim to contain "natural ingredients". It is also noted that flavoring ingredients are regulated somewhat differently:

Substances that impart flavors that have been derived from a plant or animal source may be claimed to be "natural". As well, any additive, such as preservatives and solvents added to a flavor preparation to have a technological effect solely on the flavor, does not modify the "natural" status of the flavoring material itself. However, the addition does alter the natural status of the food to which it has been added, even though it need not be declared as an ingredient on the food label... Furthermore, acids, bases, salts and sweeteners may be used to impart sour, bitter, salty and sweet tastes in conjunction with natural flavors. They do not alter the "natural" status of the flavoring material itself. - CFIA 2016

This means that although a food may not be considered "natural" by definition, the classifications of "natural ingredients" and "natural flavors" are much easier to achieve.

While these recent guidelines are careful to nail down the true definition of natural foods, the current state of the food industry makes that difficult to do, and there is still a fair amount of room for varying interpretations. The CFIA reports that these words are still often over-used and misused on labels, and advertisements, including the use of trademark names. Canadian labeling laws have their own set of complications, but importing foods and the various international laws that accompany them can complicate the issue even further.

It is safe to assume that food labels are not a reliable indicator of the true nutritional value of food choices. As a general rule, any food that comes in a package, especially if accompanied by a complicated label filled with vague terms and descriptions, should be limited or avoided. Thankfully, buying predominantly fresh foods and very minimal packaged foods can help to take the frustration and risk out of reading food labels.

3

Shopping for Health:
The Benefits of Locally Grown and Organic
Foods

Buying locally produced food is perhaps the best way to ensure healthier and higher quality food sources, while also supporting the health of the environment and the local economy.

Although it does take a little bit more care and mindfulness, the benefits of locally grown foods are certainly worth the effort. When food is produced to travel long distances before consumption, it is usually harvested long before it is fully ripe and has had the chance to reach its full nutritional potential. It is then manually ripened, using methods like ethylene gas, rather than naturally ripening on a tree or vine to receive the full spectrum of nutrients that it would normally attain throughout its lifecycle. To make matters worse, nutrient loss begins the moment a fruit or vegetable is picked. This decline continues throughout travel and its time on grocery store shelves.

Coming from smaller producers, with shorter distances to travel and much less spoilage and nutrient loss, local food is often fresher, tastier, and healthier. The difference in quality can be astounding. (Anyone who has tasted a fresh, locally grown strawberry will understand this.) Below are some tips to eating locally grown, more sustainable and healthier foods.

Visit your local farmers' markets

Farmers' markets are great places to address almost all of your needs at once. There are often several different local vendors and types of products to choose from, including local produce, meats, eggs, honey, baked goods, teas, floral arrangements, soaps, hand-made jewelry and other crafts. These open, lively environments provide an enjoyable shopping experience with an opportunity to meet and speak with local producers about their products and the methods that they use. It's also a fantastic way to connect with your community while also supporting small, hardworking farms and strengthening your local economy.

Find a trusted local farm

Take the opportunity to speak with local farmers and ask them about what they do. How far away is their farm? What types of crops do they grow? Do they use any special sustainability practices? Do they use any pesticides or other chemicals? Do they have an organic certification or use organic practices? Many local farmers may use methods that exceed organic standards, but cannot pay for an expensive organic certification. This makes their finished products even healthier than imported organic products, yet much less expensive. Once you get to know some of the farms and distributors in your area, you may choose to buy from them directly. There are some farms that may also allow customers to visit and place orders with them directly, allowing you to save money while also confirming factors like cleanliness, quality, and ethical standards.

Find local food at grocery stores

If you can't make it to a farmer's market or prefer the convenience of larger grocery stores, locally grown items can usually be found there as well. Produce items will almost always list a country, province or state of origin on the product or tag. Depending on the store and the time of year, there may even be a section in the produce department dedicated to your local area, province or county.

Grow your own food

Growing your own vegetables, fruits and herbs is an excellent step toward favorable physical, environmental, financial and mental health. During a time when the food supply seems tainted and out of our control, gardening is likely the simplest and most effective response. Caring for plants has several amazing health benefits as well, including improved air quality, mental clarity, mood regulation and physical exercise. There is a wide range of possibilities, from potted plants and small gardens at home to rented space at a community garden. Different types of urban gardens are gaining popularity as easy, healthy and affordable food sources, and as powerful cleansers for the air and environment that help to offset the effects of pollution. Food can be grown almost anywhere, including rooftops and balconies using pots, vines, and hanging baskets. Some plants are easier than others to grow and care for; for example, tomatoes, zucchini, strawberries, blueberries, potatoes, peas, cabbage and kale. Good quality seeds are fairly inexpensive and can usually be found at markets and health food stores.

Eat with the seasons

Consuming local food that is currently in season can provide endless benefits. This will allow you to eat locally and affordably while also staying in physical harmony with a changing environment. How could you go wrong when eating the foods in your own surroundings that are growing and adapting to the same conditions? Until fairly recently, all human beings and their ancestors ate this way. It's no coincidence that light, cooling, watery fruits and vegetables like berries, cherries, peppers, cucumbers, and leafy greens are in season during the hot summer months. These "expansive" fresh fruits and vegetables are helpful for cooling the body and support healthy breakdown, elimination, and detoxification. On the other hand, eating some heavier, warmer and starchier foods, such as root vegetables, meat, dairy, eggs, beans and grains, available during the winter, typically support the human body living in cold conditions. These are known more as "contractive" foods that help the body to build warmth and strength. There is something so beautiful and energetically nourishing about consuming the foods that are growing in your surrounding environment during the same season, from the same earth, using the same air and water.

Preserving some of the local food for consumption year-round is another valuable asset. Whether you are growing your own food or buying from other local sources, the use of cold cellars, fermenting, drying, canning, blanching and freezing can be very useful in preserving healthy local foods for consumption during their off-seasons.

If possible, buy organic

With more and more information and research available, there are few reasons to doubt that consuming organically grown foods is often much better for our health than those that are conventionally grown. The use of pesticides and other substances in farming methods have been associated with risks to both human and environmental health. Many of these substances are known carcinogens, neurotoxins or hormone disruptors, linked to a variety of cancers and other illnesses. Most of them are still technically legal, or are assumed by some to be present at such a low level that they won't likely cause any immediate, measurable harm. Although for a growing number of consumers, this risk doesn't seem worth it. A study from 2015 has highlighted some important differences between organic and conventional food regarding pesticide exposure. The largest of its kind so far, this study examined dietary exposure to 14 organophosphate pesticides (OPs), and assessed the influence of consuming organic produce on this exposure. Organophosphates are one of the most commonly used insecticides and have been linked to nervous system toxicity and neurological effects, as well as some types of cancer in humans who are exposed. It has been found that more frequent consumers of organic foods show significantly lower levels of OP residues in their urine than conventional consumers do. Buying organic foods is likely an important step in avoiding or reducing exposure to these organophosphates and other harmful pesticides.

Apart from pesticides used on our conventional foods, we have also been exposed to more and more genetically modified food crops (GMOs), which are a growing concern. In Britain, and throughout Europe, such food products must be clearly labeled so that the consumer can make a clear choice. It is important to recognize that adulterated, modified foods may not have the same short and long-term benefits, if any at all, compared to the healing properties of organic foods. This is often true for common genetically modified crops such as corn and soy, which exhibit clear nutritional differences from their organic counterparts. It is estimated that over 80 percent of soy products may now contain genetically altered materials. Unfortunately, genetically altered and hormone enhanced foods are considered potential hazards to our health.

While several European countries have banned or insisted on the labeling of these types of foods, many other science and government organizations have yet to reach a clear consensus on the issue. Part of the reason is that long-term multi-generational studies have not been done on humans with these foods. Having "insufficient evidence" of harmful effects is hardly enough reason to consider modified foods safe for entire populations to unknowingly consume, especially when those effects have not been sufficiently investigated. A "wait and see" approach seems like a potentially dangerous and irresponsible way to handle the health of citizens. However, as with many other public health issues, the financial interests of large corporations are an important factor. Unfortunately, there are influential companies that profit from the widespread use of controversial farming practices, making it much more difficult to ensure the safety of our food supply.

The best ways to address these concerns involve using both your voice and your buying power. Speak to your local, state or provincial and federally elected representatives and ask them what they are going to do, and what specific actions they will take on behalf of your community. While not yet legally required in North America, many companies are making the choice to refrain from using genetically modified materials in their products. Buying certified organic or non-GMO food products (indicated by official labels), sends a message to both corporations and governments about consumer demand, values and needs that should be addressed. While it seems like economic forces may be out of our control, it's important to remember that the consumer is often the most powerful force in any market.

The Dirty Dozen and the Clean Fifteen

Organic foods are often much safer and healthier; however, they can also be more expensive and harder to come by. If buying organic is a challenge, there are ways to shop with more discernment. Thankfully, there are guidelines such as those proposed by the Environmental Working Group (EWG) that allow for more educated and informed shopping choices regarding organic versus conventional produce.

The EWG's *Shopper's Guide to Pesticides in Produce* is based on results from thousands of samples that are tested by the U.S. Department of Agriculture and the Food and Drug Administration. The guide ranks pesticide contamination levels of 48 different fruits and vegetables, and creates a list of the twelve "dirtiest" and the fifteen "cleanest" fruits and vegetables on grocery shelves. The following list is updated annually in order to keep consumers up to date on the products that are most important to buy organic, and those that are less risky when grown conventionally. When opting for conventionally grown foods, even if it is listed as one of the "cleanest", a high-quality fruit and vegetable wash is useful to ensure lower amounts of residues on the surface of your produce.

2016 - The EWG's Shoppers Guide to Pesticides in Produce

The Dirty Dozen	The Clean 15
Strawberries	Avocados
Apples	Sweet Corn
Nectarines	Pineapples
Peaches	Cabbages
Celery	Sweet Peas (Frozen)
Grapes	Onions
Cherries	Asparagus
Spinach	Mangoes
Sweet Bell Peppers	Papaya
Cherry Tomatoes	Kiwi
Cucumbers	Egg Plant
Tomatoes	Honeydew Melon
	Grapefruits
	Cantaloupe
	Cauliflower

Grocery Shopping Tips

1. Do not go shopping on an empty stomach. If hungry, you may be more tempted to impulse buy items, including less-than-healthy options like processed foods.

2. Create a grocery list and stick to a budget in order to avoid overspending or making impulsive choices.

3. While shopping in most grocery stores, stick to the outside isles of the store, where most of the fresh fruits and vegetables are located, rather than the middle aisles, where there are mainly packaged and processed foods (see diagram).

4. Try to make the majority of your purchases from fresh fruits and vegetables, with smaller amounts of meat, grains and dairy.

5. Ensure that your shopping list varies week to week in terms of types and colours of fruits and vegetables to provide a full spectrum of nutrients.

6. If you must buy some packaged foods, be sure to read the label and stick to those with only whole food ingredients.

7. Avoid purchasing foods marketed as "low-fat", "fat-free", "sugar free" and "low calorie", etc.

8. Try to buy locally sourced foods whenever possible.

9. Buy organic if possible, especially for foods that have higher concentrations of pesticide residues when conventionally grown (as shown in the "The Dirty Dozen" column above).

FRESH PRODUCE

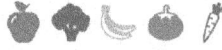

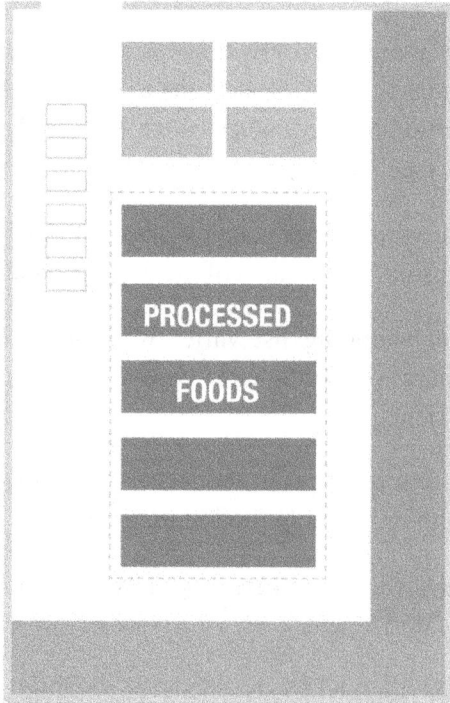

MEAT AND
SEAFOOD

PROCESSED

FOODS

EGGS AND DAIRY

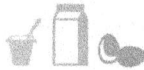

4

Making Healthy Choices Away from Home

Most of us today live fast-paced, demanding and social lifestyles, and it may not always be possible to maintain full control over what and where we are eating.

Buying raw ingredients and preparing our own food is the most effective way to ensure a fresh and nutritious diet. It's important to be mindful of where our food comes from and what is going into it. However, in the midst of traveling, hectic schedules and social engagements, it's not uncommon to find ourselves eating away from home. Luckily, there are several different ways to ensure that eating out won't completely destroy our efforts to live a healthy lifestyle.

Looking in all the right places

It may seem that when eating out, large restaurant chains and popular fast food joints are the only options. This presents obvious difficulties when trying to make healthy choices, as these menus are often filled with preservatives, salt, sugar and other not-so-fresh ingredients. Within such large chains, food is often made to travel long distances and be stored for a period of time, using freezing or additives. It can be difficult to decipher which choices are healthier than others, and sometimes the seemingly "healthy" items, such as salads, have the most concerning nutritional information. Nonetheless, while these large restaurant chains are usually the most recognizable and the most prevalent in busy areas, there are often cleaner and healthier options nearby.

When looking for fast, affordable and nutritious food, you can usually rely on health food stores, plant-based restaurants, smoothie bars or various ethnic cuisines. Steadily increasing in prevalence, health food stores will often have several nutritious, whole food meal or snack bars with adequate protein, fibre, omega fatty acids and vegetable servings. There are also different types of packaged snacks or trail mixes that are packed with nutrients and free of preservatives, although close attention should be paid to the ingredient labels. Some health food stores may even have salad bars with a variety of fresh leafy greens, seeds, oils and protein sources to choose from.

Smoothie and juice bars are other excellent spots for a quick and very nutrient-dense fix that can be taken on the go. Some options may be more filling and energizing than others, and there are several different options available for different needs, ranging from simple green juices to fuel-packed, high protein smoothies with plenty of healthy fats and fibre. When looking for fast and healthy food, you can rarely go wrong with plant-based restaurants. With menus full of fresh vegetables, there are often dozens of quick, clean salads, rice bowls, smoothies and more to choose from. However, even when choosing from seemingly healthy menus, it is important to read ingredients or ask questions to ensure that these foods are made with healthy oils and minimal added sugars or preservatives.

Sticking to certain types of cuisines are also helpful in narrowing down the search for quick and healthy food. For example, there are increasing numbers of small, family owned restaurants with different types of traditional ethnic cuisines that are quick, affordable, simple and nutritious. Many of these traditional dishes tend to be much cleaner and perhaps more flavorful than the typical North American burger and fries. For instance, many Middle Eastern and Greek restaurants tend to encompass ingredients like rice, hummus, vegetables, chickpeas, lentils and fresh salads, using simpler dressings and sauces like tahini, garlic, olive oil and lemon juice. Many of these traditional foods will also incorporate valuable spices with a wide array of health benefits, many of which may not be recognized or widely used in standard North American cooking. Various Asian cuisines will often consist of similarly clean and fresh elements, including rice, rice noodles, seaweed, fresh fish, tofu, avocado, sprouts and an array of other fresh vegetables. There are also an increasing numbers of Mexican fast food restaurants that have some high fibre, vegetable-dense options like black bean burritos, along with greens, fresh salsa and avocado. As with any other foods, it is important to use your discretion and look for options that are not heavily fried or full of harmful fats and sugars.

Local Restaurants

Another emerging trend is that of exclusively "local" restaurants, meaning that they will only use ingredients that are in season and are harvested or produced within a close radius. Choosing these types of restaurants will allow you to continue eating fresh and seasonal food. There will also be a much greater variety of foods to choose from, as the ingredients and menus will change seasonally and based on availability. It's worth considering that smaller, local businesses will also buy smaller quantities of food more often, which travel shorter distances. Some will even let their customers know if they use any organic or non-GMO ingredients. Therefore, it is almost guaranteed that you'll be consuming much fresher, less contaminated food that is in line with the climate you're currently living in. Along with these health benefits comes the knowledge that you are supporting small local businesses, as well as local farmers, and strengthening both your sense of community and the local economy as a result.

Healthy Tips for Any Restaurant

There will undoubtedly be times when you find yourself at an eating establishment that you have not carefully chosen based on your own nutritional needs and this is perfectly OK. While the skill of choosing healthy food sources is important, so is the skill of being flexible and adapting to conditions that may not be in your control. Thankfully, there are options at most restaurants that allow you to eat fairly healthy, balanced meals, and many will accommodate individual needs.

Below are some tips that will aid in making the healthiest menu selections possible.

Stick to simpler dishes with more whole food, nutrient-dense ingredients like vegetables and less sauces, dressings, and processed ingredients.

Avoid common offenders, such as refined or "white" grains, fried and breaded food, heavy sauces and glazes and excessive amounts of cheese.

This can be a critical step in reducing empty calories, the tendency to overeat and other potentially health-damaging effects. For example, a baked salmon fillet with steamed vegetables is a much more nutritious and well-rounded meal than a pasta dish with white noodles, and a cream or cheese-based sauce. You may even ask your server to leave out added sauces from some meals. Certain sauces may be more problematic than others, but these toppings often introduce a surprising amount of added fats, sugar, salt and synthetic ingredients.

When possible, ask about substituting certain ingredients with healthier alternatives. For example, heavy, additive-filled, pre-made dressings and sauces can be replaced with a fresher alternative, such as tomato sauce, olive oil and vinegar, or lemon juice. Many restaurants may also have multiple types of breads, pastas and pizza crusts to choose from, including whole-grain options, or vegetable substitutes. Sides are often interchangeable as well, including healthier options like raw or sautéed vegetables, or salads. If you're unsure about your options, ask your server for dressings or sauces on the side and use them sparingly at your own will.

The Art of Balance

In all honesty, it may not always be possible to make "perfect" choices, and you are certainly not obligated to do so. Balance is a crucial aspect of maintaining a truly healthy lifestyle, and that may include occasionally indulging in foods that are less than perfect. Most often we worry about eating unhealthy foods, but developing an unhealthy obsession with eating only "healthy" foods can be equally damaging.

As fitness and diet trends continue to gain momentum, it seems that patterns of obsessive wholesome eating are increasing as well. Also known as "orthorexia", this obsession is another form of unhealthy eating. Just like any other eating disorder, this fixation interferes with mental, social and physical health, and is ironically counterproductive to reaching the end goal. The association of fear, stress or guilt surrounding eating choices is far too common, and it is anything but healthy. In fact, mental and physical stress while eating, whether the food is considered to be "healthy" or not, can have a more significant effect on health than the food itself.

It's important to keep in mind that there is not one static definition of "health" or one distinct path to get there. Health is not a task to be achieved or a burden to carry around. It's a sensation that coincides with respecting and nourishing oneself physically, mentally, and spiritually. The meaning of health may change from person to person, moment to moment. Therefore, the most important rule to follow for optimal nutrition is to listen attentively to the needs of your own body. This doesn't mean giving in to every impulse or craving, but rather choosing the foods that will best support the body, mind and spirit in whatever state they may be in at the moment. For example, on cold days, you may gravitate toward warm, comforting soups or stews. If you have just exercised particularly hard, you might feel the need to consume more calories. And if you find yourself at a gathering with family and friends where your foods of choice aren't available, it may be in your best interest to relax and enjoy what is available. There won't always be a standard set of rules to follow, because your needs will likely fluctuate depending on several different factors.

Ultimately, food is meant to provide the energy and nutrients required for your body to function optimally. The key is to make sure that the large majority of your food choices are nourishing and energizing, rather than working against your health. For some, that majority may be 99 percent. Sometimes it might be 60 percent. Some days, it's not a majority at all. Thankfully, the human body is extremely resilient and can be forgiving. This means that no diet or lifestyle habit needs to be permanent, but it also means that even the smallest positive change will be beneficial. Regardless of what your diet looked like last month, last week or even this morning, a healthy choice can be made at any moment and your body will thank you for it.

PART II

Dietary Essentials for Optimal Health

"Let food be thy medicine and medicine be thy food."
– Hippocrates

We know that food fuels our bodies, and if eaten as fresh as possible, in the right quantity, and in harmony with our body's needs, optimal health is experienced. We have more energy, our ideal body weight is maintained and chronic diseases are kept at bay.

It can be easy to recognize whole foods that are likely to improve overall health. However, it may be more challenging to determine what it is that makes whole foods so healthy: the fatty acids, fibre, proteins, carbohydrates, micronutrients, enzymes and phytochemicals that make up these foods. It's important to know that these dietary essentials are part and parcel of consuming whole foods. They are the building blocks that give whole foods their power.

With so much information available about "healthy" foods, we are often left asking some questions: What is it that makes these foods healthy? How do we know which elements are truly nutritious and which ones are not? Will these foods still be considered healthy next month or next year? These important questions will be answered in this section of the book. Awareness of the essential nutritional fundamentals is an important step in identifying and selecting healthy foods on an ongoing basis. Rather than gathering information about which foods are healthy, knowing what makes each food healthy (or unhealthy), and how it impacts health can allow you to make informed choices suited to your own wellbeing.

Avoiding unhealthy processed foods and consuming naturally nutritious foods are great first steps. However, balance and variety are crucial. There are several key nutrients that are imperative for optimal health, and each food contains different combinations and amounts of these nutrients. For maintenance and prevention, it's important to ensure that your food choices are covering all of the necessary bases that are outlined in the following chapters.

Of course, each individual is biochemically unique, and therefore, may have slightly different nutritional needs. Accordingly, if you are hoping to address a particular illness, imbalance or goal, we suggest working with a practitioner who can assess your specific needs and make recommendations accordingly.

5

Essential Fats & Oils

Fats are often given a bad rap, but the truth is that you cannot live without them.

In past decades, dietary fat has often been feared by both consumers and experts – perhaps due to its high caloric value, or its poorly understood association with the fat that is deposited in unwanted places in the body. However, more recent research shows that adequate fat intake is crucial to preventing many common diseases; for instance, premenstrual syndrome, menopausal symptoms, infertility, arthritis, psoriasis and eczema, cardiovascular disease, attention deficit disorders, and multiple sclerosis. As it turns out, healthy fat intake is also important for healthy weight management, and the reduction of stored fat. Physicians and researchers are discovering that by optimizing the blend of dietary oils, they can positively change the body's supply of beneficial prostaglandins, optimize several physiological functions, and in some cases, treat disease.

It has been estimated that the typical North American diet only provides 20 percent of the essential fatty acids required for optimal function and health. Unfortunately, a lack of the right fats often leads to systemic imbalances, which inevitably lead to many illnesses. Another part of the equation is that other influences, such as alcohol and caffeine consumption, chemical exposure, air pollution, drug use and a stressful lifestyle, easily deplete fatty acids, only adding to the problem. Many common foods are also filled with *unhealthy* fats that can be extremely damaging to several body systems. The key is moderation and a balance of different types of high-quality fats consumed on a regular basis.

Why are good fats necessary?

Healthy fat intake is required for several functions. Your body needs fat for energy, metabolism and storage of fat-soluble vitamins (Vitamins A, D, E and F), and healthy hormone production. It is also required for development and structure. In fact, your brain is composed mainly of fat – about 65 percent. Your nerves are protected with an outer layer of fat, as is the entire body. This aspect of structure is critical to communication between cells, temperature maintenance, isolation of harmful substances and energy storage. One gram of this storage is nine calories of banked energy, just waiting to be released. It takes very little energy to maintain fat, whereas muscle requires and uses much more energy to maintain itself, even when you are at rest. Healthy fat intake, and the individual fatty acids that fat provides, contribute to almost every physiological function in some way.

What are the different types of fats?

Naturally occurring fats are either classified as saturated, polyunsaturated or monounsaturated. Saturated fats, which are more stable than unsaturated oils, are mainly found in sources like animal fats with the exception of coconut or palm oils. Due to their stability, these fats are often more desirable for cooking, because they can withstand higher heats without being chemically altered. Conversely, unsaturated oils increase fluidity and flexibility, easily moving apart. Mono-and polyunsaturated fats are mainly found in plant and fish sources, with a reputation for numerous health benefits.

The body is able to manufacture some of the fats that it needs, with the exception of two important polyunsaturated fatty acids: omega-3 and omega-6, called essential fatty acids, due to the fact that they must come from our foods. Consuming these fats in the correct ratio is vital in determining how well the body is able to function.

Essential Fatty Acids (EFAs), sometimes referred to as Vitamin F, are some of the most important nutritional components found in dietary fats and oils. Crucial to optimal health, they are responsible for the following important tasks:

- Transportation and metabolism of blood triglycerides and cholesterol. EFAs are shown to greatly reduce the levels of these substances when they have become too high
- Optimizing several functions by increasing metabolic rate, energy production and oxygen uptake
- Contribute to cell membrane flexibility, fluidity and selective permeability by allowing crucial products into cells and keeping harmful ones out
- Maintaining and enhancing normal brain development and functioning
- Manufacturing of eicosanoids, including hormone-like substances called prostaglandins that regulate critical functions, such as arterial muscle tone, the transport of oxygen in the blood, sodium excretion through the kidneys, inflammatory response and immune system functions

These functions translate to countless benefits and implications for overall health:

- Prevention of heart disease, stroke and diabetes
- Essential for the central nervous system and promotes healthy nerve activity
- Aids in vitamin absorption, especially fat-soluble vitamins
- Maintains a healthy immune system
- Helps to promote cell development
- Insulates cells membranes crucial for brain, eyes and skin

Of the essential fatty acids consumed by average North Americans, the majority of them tend to be omega-6 fatty acids. This is thought to be due to an overreliance on vegetable oils that are rich in omega-6, along with reduced consumption of fresh fish. While adequate omega-6 intake is important, most people require much more omega-3 essential fatty acids in order to maintain a balanced ratio.

Omega-3 Fatty Acids

Omega-3 is an especially essential family of unsaturated fatty acids that has important roles in health. The National Institutes of Health (NIH) reported that the majority of US diets no longer contain the amount of omega-3 fatty acids needed by our bodies.

Types of omega-3 fatty acids include:

- Alpha Linolenic Acid (ALA) - found in flax and hemp oil
- Eicosapentaenoic Acid (EPA) - found in fish oil
- Docosahexaenois Acid (DHA) - found in fish oil
- Linoleic Acid (LA) - found in flax, hemp, borage and evening primrose oils
- Gamma Linolenic Acid (GLA) - found in borage oil, hemp oil and evening primrose oil

Two of the most important types of long chain omega-3 fatty acids include eicosapentaenoic acid (EPA), and docosahexaenoic acid (DHA). These fatty acids are critical for the production of nerve tissue, hormones, and cellular membranes. Both can be synthesized from alpha-linoleic acid (ALA); however, this conversion is believed to be inefficient in most people. EPA is found to maintain and support cardiovascular health, inflammatory reduction and healthy skin, whereas DHA is best known for supporting the development of the brain, eyes and nerves. With membrane-enhancing capabilities in brain cells, DHA is essential for the proper function of our brains as adults and for the development of our nervous system and visual abilities during pregnancy and the first six months of life.

Sources of omega-3 fatty acids include fish like salmon, sardines and mackerel, as well as some plant sources, such as hemp seeds, walnuts, chia seeds, flax seeds and marine algae. However, it's worth noting that we likely do not actually convert very much omega-3 fatty acids from nuts and seeds compared to omega-6. Therefore, if fish consumption is low, it's important to make sure that fish oils or other omega-3 supplements like algae are consumed in order to maintain adequate levels.

Omega-6 Fatty Acids

Omega-6 fatty acids, like omega-3, are essential for human health, and cannot be made by the human body. They also play an essential role in brain function and normal growth development. This polyunsaturated fatty acid helps to stimulate skin, hair and bone health, and maintain the reproductive system. Sources include seeds, nuts and vegetable oils, providing mainly linoleic acid (LA). LA can be converted to gamma-linolenic acid (GLA), which is found in evening primrose oil, borage oil and black currant seed oil. Because the standard North American diet is abundant in omega-6 fatty acids, you can reduce omega-6 levels by eating less processed and fast foods, and polyunsaturated vegetable oils, such as corn, sunflower, safflower, soy and cottonseed. Instead, focus on consuming a blend of healthier, more balanced fats that comprise of both omega-3 and omega-6 sources.

Omega-9 Fatty Acids

The omega-9 monounsaturated fatty acid can be synthesized by the body and is therefore categorized as "non-essential". It is found in olive oil, peanut oil, sunflower oil, avocados, olives, almonds, pecans, walnuts and pistachios. Its "non-essential" nature means that we do not depend solely on our foods for this type of omega fatty acid. Focusing on the limited and essential types, such as omega-3, is generally more important in maintaining a healthy balance. However, omega-9 fatty acids are still important for many similar aspects of health.

What is Cholesterol?

Cholesterol is a unique type of fat. As an essential compound, it is synthesized internally and is a key component of cell membranes. Cholesterol is a lipid-like, waxy alcohol that is transported in the blood plasma and is required to maintain proper membrane permeability and fluidity. Found primarily in animal fats, blood, nerve tissue and bile, 66 to 85 percent of needed cholesterol is produced by the liver or intestines.

48

Cholesterol has many benefits and is critical for the following:

- Carbohydrate metabolism
- Helping the skin convert the sun's ultraviolet rays into essential Vitamin D
- Vital component of cell membranes
- The main supplier of steroid hormones; for example, cortisone and various sex hormones.

However, cholesterol is known to have a good and bad side. While minimum levels of cholesterol are essential for life, excess levels in the bloodstream indicate a buildup and possible blockage of blood vessels, and are correlated with increased cardiovascular diseases (CVD), which are the leading causes of morbidity and mortality in Europe and North America.

Canadian statistics mention that CVD accounts for the death of more Canadians than any other disease. According to WHO research, high cholesterol may be linked to more than half (56 percent), of all cases of coronary heart disease worldwide, and is linked to about 4.4 million deaths per year. In recent decades, researchers have investigated the effects of elevated serum cholesterol levels as a risk factor that can be modified to prevent heart disease. As a result, many people fear dietary cholesterol as a contributor to high cholesterol levels and increased risk of cardiovascular disease.

However, newer findings have painted a much clearer picture of the relationship between cholesterol and cardiovascular disease. It appears that cholesterol levels and CVD risk are likely both affected by factors such as refined sugar consumption, stress and other influences like smoking and alcohol consumption that cause oxidative damage and inflammation, rather than by dietary cholesterol intake. This is because in addition to what we eat, our bodies produce significant quantities of cholesterol, typically much more than we get from our diets. Simply put: when arteries and blood vessels are damaged by harmful forces like sugar, stress, alcohol and drug use, the body uses cholesterol as a mechanism to repair or "patch" the damaged areas. Over time, and combined with a lack of nutrients that support healing and excretion of excess cholesterol, this will likely lead to higher than normal levels of LDL cholesterol in the blood, as well as cholesterol deposits, blockages, hardening of the arteries and cardiovascular disease.

Since cholesterol is insoluble in the blood, it is transported in the circulatory system within lipoproteins. Low density lipoproteins (LDLs) are the major transporters of cholesterol in the blood stream and, because LDLs seem to encourage the deposit of cholesterol in the arteries, it is also known as "bad" cholesterol. Arteriosclerosis begins with changes in the endothelial cell function, and having elevated LDL levels is one of the major risk factors contributing to this process. When the cardiovascular system is not properly functioning, and there are elevated levels of LDL, plaque is formed that sticks to the artery walls and is regarded as atherogenic: prone to cause atherosclerosis. On the other hand, high density lipoproteins (HDLs) are considered to be "good" cholesterol because they carry unneeded cholesterol away from the cells and back to the liver, where it is broken down for removal from the body, resulting in better health.

Blood tests for cholesterol usually include measuring blood triglyceride levels. High triglyceride levels do not mean you will have high cholesterol readings. Low triglyceride levels do not mean you will have low cholesterol readings. It does appear, however, that if you manage to lower your triglyceride levels, your cholesterol levels will fall as well.

Modern science has found a better test predictor for your cardiovascular system health status: testing for elevated levels of the amino acid homocysteine. There are many natural approaches and supplements that can help to normalize these levels, including the consumption of a variety of nutrients and phytonutrients with antioxidant activity. Healthcare practitioners have also used high doses of Vitamins B6, B12 and folic acid, and sometimes B3 (niacin), to successfully reduce homocysteine levels.

Table 1 below shows the risk categories and target lipid levels.

Risk category	LDL-C level mmol/L	TC:HDL-C ratio
High* (10-year risk of coronary artery Disease - 20%, or history of diabetes mellitus** or any atherosclerotic disease)	<2.5 and	< 4.0
Moderate (10-year risk 11%–19%)	< 3.5 and	< 5.0
Low*** (10-year risk 10%)	< 4.5 and	< 6.0

Source: CMAJ • 28 OCT. 2003; 169 (9)

The American Heart Association provides a similar set of guidelines for total (fasting) blood cholesterol levels and risk for heart disease. The desirable LDL level is considered to be less than 100 mg/dL (2.6 mmol)

Eventually, if one has elevated LDL cholesterol, they can exhibit certain symptoms, such as a faint pulse in the lower extremities, neurasthenia, angina pain, leg cramps, trembling and shortness of breath. Aside from elevated LDL cholesterol, there are many other associated risk factors that can contribute to cardiovascular disease.

The Risk of Consuming Unhealthy Fats

Consuming enough healthy fats is clearly a very important aspect of overall health. However, this is only a small part of the story. When you consume unhealthy fats, not only will it contribute to unwanted weight gain, but it will likely impact several other aspects of health as well.

The last hundred years have seen a massive increase in cardiovascular disease and cancer in Western cultures. A major change has occurred in our diets, including certain oils that did not exist until the latter half of the 20[th]century, which means we have not evolved long enough to know the exact long-term side effects on our health. Changing diets, food processing methods, and technological manipulations without sufficient long-term studies, are leading to a healthcare crisis among many people, both young and old.

Trans fats are one type of common manmade fat that is generally suspected as a contributor to many illnesses. These fatty acids are often created during the production of processed, packaged and fast foods. They come hidden in common oils and foods, such as French fries, margarine, ice creams, donuts, corn chips, potato chips, and the vast majority of chemically altered and processed foods. The main benefit of trans-fatty acids is to extend the shelf life of a product. Unfortunately, it may decrease the length and quality of your life at the same time.

This volume of synthetically made trans-fatty acids did not exist a hundred years ago. Evolutionary biology is uncovering the partnership that slowly evolved between humankind and the earth over thousands of generations, possibly millions of years. We can change our environment, but can our minds and bodies adapt and adjust to these changes at the same speed? The answer is no. This is evidenced by increasing amounts of cardiovascular diseases, cancers and attention deficit disorders in Western societies.

Every cell in the human body needs fat to continue the process of cell regeneration. Cell membranes are greatly affected by the types of fats that they are given to grow and thrive. While healthy mono-and polyunsaturated fats often increase the strength of the cell, certain saturated fats and trans-fatty acids instead hinder the growth of healthy cell membranes. Each organ and structure in the body is simply a collection of cells. This means that unhealthy fat intake, causing damage and deficiency at a cellular level, is sure to disrupt internal organ function and overall physical health.

What makes a fat or oil unhealthy?

While some fats are more stable than others, there are some conditions that no nutrient can successfully withstand. Processing at high temperatures destroys several beneficial components of many oils and alters the chemical structure, creating much more harmful substances. The use of preservatives, chemical solvents, high temperatures and even exposure to excessive sunlight, are all major threats to the healthy properties of unsaturated fats. During the production of shortening, margarine and the vast majority of processed foods, vegetable oils are often altered to create hydrogenated or partially hydrogenated fats, which result in the production of trans fats – the main suspects in disease and illness when it comes to fats.

Naturally occurring fatty acids are usually easily recognized and utilized by the human body; however, these permanently altered structures are not. Studies indicate that the consumption of trans-fatty acids is a major factor associated with many types of cancer and heart disease. They have been proven to lower the levels of the good cholesterol (HDL) and increase the levels of bad cholesterol (LDL), throwing off the balance needed between the two for optimal health. In addition, they create problems with your body's ability to utilize and properly metabolize the essential fatty acids.

Sources of toxic fats and oils

Hidden fats in the foods we eat are often the most harmful and are very different substances than the essential fats we need for optimal health and healing. In the 1940s, grocery stores generally had 300 to 400 food items and relatively few were processed. Today, the average supermarket has between 30,000 and 50,000 items, most of which are processed. It is these processed foods that contain the potentially damaging fats.

These foods include classically "unhealthy" foods, including meat products like hot dogs, hamburgers and cold cuts, as well as cakes, donuts, candies, ice creams and French fries. However, most packaged foods in general, even those that may be promoted as healthier alternatives, often come laced with unhealthy fats. The cheap fats that are used during processing are refined, deodorized and usually hydrogenated to prolong shelf life, becoming oxidized or rancid.

High temperature frying changes the chemical composition of essential fatty acids into toxic substances that affect your health over time. All vegetable oils that are hydrogenated or partially hydrogenated should be avoided. Read the labels, and if dining out, ask to see the type of fats and oils they use. Here are the top three oils used in commercially made products:

- **Cottonseed oil**. Cotton is one of the most heavily sprayed crops. It contains man-made and natural toxins. The fast food industry extensively uses this inexpensive toxic oil.
- **Corn oil.** Toxic solvents and high temperatures are usually used during processing. As a result, most widely used, commercial grades become rancid. If using corn oil, look for organically grown cold pressed, mechanically processed unrefined corn oil from corn germ.
- **Soybean oil.** Due to the difficulty in extracting oil from soybeans, the oil is usually damaged in the process, using high temperatures and toxic solvents.

How are good oils made and recognized?

Expeller pressing processes quality oils at temperatures below 118 degrees Fahrenheit in light and oxygen free environments. Next, they are stored and refrigerated in amber or dark colored, light resistant containers. It is crucial that oils are protected from high heat, light and oxygen in order to avoid destruction of nutritional components or creation of harmful substances. Most healthy oils will normally be indicated as "cold-pressed", "virgin", "extra-virgin" and "unrefined". However, it's important to be careful of misleading advertising and stick to well-known companies that can be trusted.

Choosing Healthy Fats and Oils

The health and safety of oils depend mostly on the growing practices, processing techniques, and natural chemical properties of each oil. Monounsaturated and polyunsaturated oils that are liquid at room temperature are often healthy choices, as long as they are safely processed. However, many unsaturated oils are not ideal for cooking. In recent years, saturated fats have also gained a lot of recognition for their health benefits, including their higher heat stability. Popular examples include coconut oil, palm oil and ghee (clarified butter).

Cold pressed, organically grown monounsaturated fats are an excellent choice, supported by findings in the 1980s, regarding the nutritional benefits of a Mediterranean diet including pure olive oil. Other monounsaturated fats can be found in the oil from macadamia nuts, hazelnuts, walnuts, almonds, avocados and pistachios. Research on monounsaturated fats generally indicates it does not increase risk of heart disease, but too much of a good thing can lead to weight gain and imbalances, adding unnecessary additional stress on the body.

Monounsaturated fats can reduce total cholesterol while improving the ratio of the HDL (good cholesterol) to LDL (bad cholesterol), and reduce the levels of blood triglycerides. Studies show monounsaturated fatty acids can help diabetics improve control over their blood sugar levels, possibly resulting in significant reductions of the amount of insulin they require daily.

With new science available, certain types of saturated fats are gaining appreciation for their abundance of health benefits, including natural, mainly plant-based sources, such as coconut oil. It was found that they are beneficial for the proper function of several body systems, including cell membranes, liver, heart, hormones and immune system. They also remain more stable at high temperatures, making them suitable for cooking.

More specifically, medium chain triglycerides (MCTs) are gaining momentum as a great energy source, which increases athletic endurance, reduces cholesterol levels, and aids in weight loss. While this may be true, using only isolated MCT oils, and ignoring other healthy fats, may not be helpful in achieving optimal health and wellbeing long-term. Balance is key here – occasional use may be helpful, but if you deprive your body of other forms of fat or complete unrefined oils, then you may be missing out on an array of other nutritional benefits. Coconut and palm kernel oils are rich in MCTs, and as more complete, unrefined products, they may be a healthier choice for long-term, everyday use. If supplementing with MCTs, it's important to follow label directions, continue eating a balanced diet, and consult with your doctor or natural healthcare provider if you are planning on using them for prolonged periods.

How can I get the fats I need, in the right amounts?

To ensure adequate essential fatty acid intake, it is suggested to take approximately one teaspoon to one tablespoon of a cold pressed, organically produced omega-3-rich oil such as fish oil, algae oil or flax seed oil each day (depending on the strength or concentration of omega-3 fatty acids). Plant-based oils like flax or hemp or olive oils are great additions to salads and other meals (if they are hot, let them cool before adding oils).

Hemp oil is the closest to the one-to-three ratio that the body best utilizes. Next is flax seed oil, then walnut oil. In all cases, we refer to cold pressed, mechanically extracted oil only.

Good sources of omega-3 essential fatty acids include: flax oil, hemp oil, soya, herring, mackerel, salmon, sardines, shellfish and even dark green leafy vegetables.

Good sources of omega-6 essential fatty acids include: borage oil, corn oil, evening primrose oil, hemp oil, safflower oil, sesame oil, sunflower oil, beef, chicken, eggs, lamb, legumes, nuts, pork and seeds.

Spreads like margarine, while popularly known as a healthier alternative, are often hydrogenated and have been found in increase LDL cholesterol. This makes naturally saturated fats like unrefined coconut oil, organic butter or ghee much better choices.

What proportion of fats or oils should I have in my daily allowance of calories?

For an average healthy adult, it is estimated that between 15 to 20 percent of your total daily calories should come from fats and oils. This is usually between two to five tablespoons of fat or oils from all sources. Each tablespoon is roughly 120 calories. If you eat 1,500 calories a day, that means you need roughly 225 to 300 calories of good fats and oils each day. Of course, this proportion could fluctuate depending on individual needs. However, these numbers represent the recommended minimum for the average person to maintain optimal health.

Recommended Oils and Fats for Cooking

Keep in mind that heat destroys the beneficial properties of fats and oils, including omega-3 and omega-6 essential fatty acids. You can use fats and oils in baking at temperatures up to 325 degrees Fahrenheit. Boiling, deep-frying and frying alter the chemistry of oils, negatively impacting their composition in terms of beneficial health properties. If you must fry, it is preferable to use the oils with the highest saturated and monounsaturated (omega-9) fatty acids content: coconut oil, avocado oil and palm oil. It's important to cook most foods at the lowest possible heat, and watch for smoking or browning. This indicates that there is a chemical change in the oil. Below are some oils that can be great for cooking.

- *Extra Virgin Olive Oil* lasts the longest of the cold pressed oils - about two years. If frozen, it makes an excellent solid spread that quickly liquefies at room temperature. For cooking or salads, you can substitute two tablespoons for each three tablespoons of most other oils you would use, since olive oil has a rich flavour.
- *Monounsaturated oils:* Macadamia oil, hazelnut oil, almond oil, avocado oil, pistachio oil, or extra virgin olive oil
- *Ghee or Butter*
- *Tropical oils*, such as cocoa, coconut, palm and Shea butter.

Healthy Cooking Tips

- Sulphur rich foods like garlic and onions help minimize free radical damage while frying. Combine them with the oils and fats, which are recommended for cooking.
- Wok cooking is a quick frying technique, which helps reduce damage to vegetables and food compared to other methods of frying. First add water to the wok, then vegetables; then the oil. The trick is to stir frequently to prevent scorching. Use the sides of the wok for cooking. Add spices and oil mixtures after main dishes and vegetables are cooked.
- For salads and fresh vegetables, the best choice is fresh oils or seeds with the oil still in them.

Less healthy fat sources to decrease or remove from your diet:

- Margarine
- Red meat
- Nonorganic butter
- Dairy products (especially if they may have been produced using bovine growth hormones, antibiotics, or unnaturally genetically altered cows)
- Prepared luncheon and deli meats
- Processed and sweetened nut butters with additives
- Potato and corn chips
- Pastries and candy
- Fried and deep fried foods

Healthy Fat Sources to Increase
(All fresh or cold-pressed sources, if possible)

- Nuts and seeds
- Eggs
- Flax, hemp and borage oils
- Sea vegetables
- Cold water fish and fish oils
- Coconut, avocado and palm oils
- Organic butter or ghee
- Fresh organically grown vegetables and legumes

6

Carbohydrates

Carbohydrates have the potential to be both life-giving and destructive.
The difference exists in the sources and how they are consumed.

This class of molecules represents the body's quickest and most accessible sources of energy. This is because most carbohydrates are easily broken down into sugars known as glucose – a molecule that is critical for central nervous system function and energy production, fueling every action. As an extremely efficient fuel source, foods that are high in carbohydrates have likely been critical to the survival of our ancestors. With this in mind, it's easy to see why sweet tastes are so appealing. This means that you can blame your sugar cravings on evolution – but only partially.

High-carbohydrate foods are prevalent in our modern society, to say the least. However, with exponentially higher intakes and much lower activity levels, we are experiencing a dramatic imbalance when compared to our ancestors. This pattern results in a long list of health issues, including blood sugar imbalances, which create a vicious cycle as blood sugar levels spike and drop, and cravings increase.

Our cells are able to use energy from carbohydrates very quickly and effectively. This is excellent news, if your cells are starved for energy, but most people in first world countries never truly experience that state. Instead, our cells are bombarded with more and more unnecessary sugars, doing damage to almost every part of our bodies, and storing the excess energy as extra weight. To make matters worse, sugars are also used very efficiently by other forces that plague our health, including pathogenic bacteria, yeast and even some diseased cells, such as cancer.

Another major problem with modern carbohydrates is that many forms seem to have evolved into super-carbs, invading our food supply in excessive amounts. The carbohydrates that are in the majority of popular modern foods have been refined or synthesized to contain absurd amounts of sugar. Anything consumed in excess will be harmful, especially when it has been altered and refined. While carbohydrates as a whole are not dangerous, refined sugars are.

Awareness of the differences between various sources and amounts of carbohydrates is crucial, along with balance and moderation.

Types of Carbohydrates

Carbohydrates may fall into two different categories: simple and complex.

1. **Simple carbohydrates**, also known as simple sugars, include table sugar (sucrose), fruit sugar (fructose), milk sugar (lactose), and other similar individual sugar molecules.

2. **Complex carbohydrates** are sugar molecules linked together to form longer more complex chains. Foods containing complex carbohydrates include vegetables, beans, peas and whole grains, which often contain a combination of starches, and fibres.

Fibre is a particular carbohydrate of interest when it comes to nutritional wellbeing. It is the only carbohydrate that is not digestible, and cannot be changed into glucose or glycogen. However, fibre does play several important roles in digestion, metabolism and excretion.

As a tough and indigestible component of plant-based foods, fibre is crucial to digestion, detoxification, cholesterol regulation, and prevention of several diseases. It facilitates the movement of food through the digestive system, binds and isolates harmful substances for excretion, and keeps the intestinal system healthy, strong and "clean". Certain types of fibre even nourish healthy intestinal bacteria, which will be explained in an upcoming chapter.

Benefits of Fibre:

- Lowers blood pressure
- Contributes to healthy cholesterol levels
- Stabilizes blood sugar levels

- Maintains healthy gut ecology (bacterial cultures)
- Reduces tendencies to overeat by increasing satiety (the sensation of fullness)
- Facilitates digestive movement and function
- Lessens the amount of time food is in the digestive tract
- Helps "scrub" the intestines, removing debris and keeping the digestive system clean

Health conditions and imbalances that can be prevented by adequate fibre include: hemorrhoids, varicose veins, gallstones, Type 2 diabetes, obesity, colitis, hormonal imbalances, premenstrual syndrome (PMS), menopausal symptoms and breast cancer, as well as a long list of digestive disturbances and disorders.

It has also been noted that increased intake of dietary fibre lowers risk for developing cardiovascular disease (CVD), stroke, hypertension, certain forms of cancer and gastrointestinal diseases.

It should be noted that increasing fibre may not be right for everyone, such as those with specific digestive disorders that could be easily aggravated. As with any specific disorders or illnesses, it's best to check with a practitioner before making any major dietary changes. There are two types of dietary fibre:

Insoluble Fibre is completely indigestible fibre or "roughage". Its key roles involve moving food through the digestive tract, increasing stool bulk, and controlling pH (acidity) levels in the intestines. Research has shown that insoluble fibre prevents constipation, accelerates toxic removal and prevents the growth of pathogenic bacteria, therefore preventing diseases, such as colorectal cancer. Sources of insoluble fibre include: whole oat or wheat bran, flax seeds, corn kernels and vegetables like leafy greens and celery.

Soluble Fibre is fibre that can be partially dissolved or broken down, making it able to form a gel that expands, binds and traps certain materials in the digestive system for excretion. As a result, soluble fibre intake is needed for healthy excretion, detoxification and cholesterol regulation.

Sources of soluble fibre include: chia seeds, beans and legumes, cauliflower, potatoes (with skin), dark green leafy vegetables, root vegetable skins, fruit skins, apple pectin, wheat bran, nuts and seeds, whole grains of wheat, barley, and rye, etc.

Daily Fibre Intake Recommendations for Adults

	Age 50 or younger	Age 51 or older
Men	38 grams	30 grams
Women	25 grams	21 grams

(Mayo Clinic)

Carbohydrate Metabolism

Carbohydrates have been blamed for an array of health issues, and for good reasons. However, it's important to understand which types of carbohydrates are harmful and how. The difference lies in metabolism.

Normally, "easy" digestion would sound pretty great. However, when carbohydrates are broken down to release glucose into the blood very quickly, in high amounts, or too often, they can do much more harm than good – wreaking havoc on blood sugar levels and insulin sensitivity, and doing damage to the brain, nerves and arteries in the process.

The rate at which carbohydrates are processed into fuel is an important factor in blood sugar regulation. This rate is measured using the **glycemic index**, which indicates a food's direct effect on blood sugar. High glycemic foods normally include those that are high in sugars and starches. The glucose derived from them rapidly enters the bloodstream, causing your pancreas to work hard to produce the insulin needed to use it and store it. This repeated assault on blood sugar and pancreas function eventually leads to blood sugar imbalances, metabolic syndrome, diabetes and associated complications.

After consuming a surplus of carbohydrates, the excess is converted from glucose into glycogen by the liver, before eventually being stored as fat. The liver stores the glucose and glycogen, converting them into fat for future energy needs. Too little carbohydrates and your body will need to use the stored glycogen, fats, and proteins for energy. This metabolic state is referred to as "ketosis", which relies mainly on body fat, dietary fat and protein as primary energy sources.

Sources of Carbohydrates

There are many natural foods that contain easily digestible sugars, and they can be extremely useful as quick energy sources to replenish glycogen stores or provide a quick boost that requires little digestive effort. These natural sugars found in foods like fruit are normally accompanied by a spectrum of other useful nutrients that aid in safe and effective metabolism. Some fruits may even be considered high glycemic, but certainly do not act in the exact same way as white bread. Natural or "whole" sources of sugar like fruit will have appropriate amounts of sugar, and will generally be digested and metabolized very well without doing any harm, as long as they are not over-consumed. It's no coincidence that many natural sources of sugar come along with valuable antioxidants, fibre and vitamins that aid in healthy sugar metabolism.

High glycemic foods like refined and processed sugars are so quickly digested that they can become dangerous. For example, refined white sugar or high-fructose corn syrup contains much higher amounts of sugars than would ever be present in nature. To make matters worse, they are also missing the fibre, amino acids and other nutrients that are needed for safe effective sugar metabolism. In contrast, naturally sweet ingredients, such as dates, pure maple syrup, or pure, unpasteurized honey can provide health benefits without sacrificing taste.

High glycemic foods to avoid or cut back on: refined white sugar, white flour breads and pastas, candies, cakes, cookies, potato chips, pretzels, soft drinks, white rice, starchy vegetables, such as potatoes or carrots, dried fruits, sweet corn, and of course, packaged foods containing added fructose, sucrose, sugar or other sweeteners.

*Note: Beware of sugar substitutes or other chemical sweeteners. While they may not be considered high glycemic, they can sometimes be even more damaging, and many still have some effect on insulin and blood sugar. Even those that are natural and low in calories should be consumed in moderation, because at the very least, they are continuing to affect sugar cravings, and add to an extremely "over-sweetened" dietary culture.

Low glycemic foods are usually higher in fibre, providing more slowly digested carbohydrates. They are generally much gentler on the pancreas, and therefore, on all other tissues in the body, providing energy in a more constant and even flow.

Your daily food intake, in terms of calories, may be up to 60 percent carbohydrates, the majority of them being complex carbohydrates and fibres. Needs are likely to significantly fluctuate based on activity level and lifestyle. Keep in mind that this amount should include the adequate amount of fibre your body needs to function at its best.

Lower glycemic carbohydrate sources: oatmeal, whole grains, sprouted breads, high fibre fruits (apples, berries, fresh oranges, apricots, mangoes, etc.), high fibre vegetables (Brussels sprouts, broccoli, onions, etc.), beans and legumes (chickpeas, mung, pinto, edamame).

7

Proteins & Amino Acids

With a long list of structural and biochemical functions, proteins, and the amino acids that they are comprised of, are fundamental to life.

Proteins are the second most abundant material, next to water, that makes up the human body. They are crucial to the structure of your muscles, tendons, ligaments, glands, organs, nails, hair and body fluids. Proteins are linked chains of amino acids, held together by peptide bonds. Each type of protein is unique in its chemical sequencing, fulfilling a specific need in the body, and is not interchangeable with any other protein. Dietary protein is broken down into its amino acid components, then reconstituted as the specific proteins your body needs at that time. So, just as dietary proteins are made up of individual amino acids, the process of protein digestion also results in the creation of distinct amino acids as end products.

The following are some of the functions proteins are involved in:

- Structure of muscle and other tissues
- Muscle and bone growth
- Brain and nervous system function
- Immunity and illness prevention
- Balance and maintenance of internal pH
- Nutrient exchange between the tissues, blood and lymph
- Part of the structural basis of genetic material

Amino acids are popularly called the 'building blocks' or the nitrogenous organic acids, that make up peptides, polypeptides and proteins. Twenty-six of the more than 100 naturally occurring amino acids are used by the body to create the proteins needed for optimal function.

Nine amino acids that are considered to be **essential** for adults:

- Histidine
- Isoleucine
- Leucine
- Lysine
- Methionine
- Phenylalanine
- Threonine
- Tryptophan
- Valine

To be "essential" means that the body cannot manufacture or produce them on its own, and therefore, must acquire them from an external source, such as breast milk, specific foods, or supplements. While the **non-essential** ones (about 80 percent) can be manufactured by the liver, all amino acids are necessary and some may even be considered "conditionally essential".

Although the human body is able to produce certain amino acids, it requires the various tools and materials necessary to do so, which may include other amino acids and micronutrients. Also, when an essential amino acid is missing or low, the capability of all the other amino acids is proportionally reduced. For these reasons, it's best to ensure a well-rounded diet containing a wide variety of vitamins, minerals and protein sources including both essential and non-essential amino acids.

The following is a list of some of the functions that amino acids are involved in:

- Act as neurotransmitters (or precursors to them)
- Some are needed for the brain to send and receive messages, and are able to pass through the blood-brain barrier
- Aid in communication with nerve cells in other parts of the body
- Allow several other nutrients to be metabolized and used more efficiently

Protein and Amino Acid Sources

The importance of dietary protein is well-known. It's crucial for body composition and structure, as well as communication between all of our cells and organ systems. However, as more information has been gathered about the roles of individual amino acids, it's clear that we must pay attention to not only the amount of protein we're consuming, but the sources and amino acid compositions of those proteins. This isn't to say that each of us should be counting our intake of dozens of different amino acids each day. Rather, it can be extremely helpful to be mindful of regularly consuming a wide variety of protein sources with complementary amino acid profiles.

Of course, amino acids are most abundant in high-protein foods, although all foods do contain some amino acids. For example, protein sources such as meats, fish, eggs and dairy have higher amounts of amino acids and are usually considered **complete proteins**, meaning that they contain all essential amino acids. On the other hand, vegan and vegetarian sources of protein are lower in certain essential amino acids, and may be classified as **incomplete proteins**. However, many of these sources do contain adequate amounts of most essential amino acids, and can be easily combined with other vegetables sources to create complete essential amino acid profiles or "complete proteins".

Ensuring a balanced diet with a variety of protein sources is the most important factor in attaining a healthy mix of amino acids. While animal foods generally contain all essential amino acids, over-consumption should be avoided for several reasons.

Those who do not eat animal foods need to be particularly mindful of their amino acid consumption. Consuming a mix of several protein-rich plant foods over time will normally do the trick, but there are certain combinations that will be sure to provide "complete" proteins. For example, combinations including whole grains along with beans, legumes or seeds will provide a good protein balance.

Supplementation

Although consuming a variety of whole food protein sources is the best way to maintain optimal health, supplementation can be useful in certain situations. For example, during periods of increased protein demands, complete protein powders made from organic whey or sprouted vegan blends can be helpful additions to complete a diet. Amino acids may also be supplemented separately for therapeutic purposes, as each individual amino acid has its own unique applications and roles in human health. There are several amino acid supplements available for various purposes, from muscle recovery to nervous system function and intestinal health. If considering amino acid supplements, it's best to speak to a trained practitioner about which ones are best for you. In general, it is recommended to rely mainly on whole food sources, and to limit and/or cycle individual supplementation as to not upset the balance of other amino acids.

8

Life-Supporting Bacteria

Maintaining the health of the body's microbial residents may be just as important as the health of our own human cells.

In recent years, most people have heard of probiotic bacteria, mainly in the context of fermented foods like yogurt or its role in digestion. In fact, beneficial bacteria have been steadily gaining recognition for its crucial roles in every single aspect of human health.

The word "probiotic" is defined by the World Health Organization as "live micro-organisms, which, when administered in adequate amounts, confer a health benefit on the host". You may have heard various statistics stating that each of us is made up of more bacterial cells than human cells. This is likely true: we are covered in bacteria, and while this may sound unsettling, it is our symbiotic relationship with these bacteria that allows us to live and function optimally. Although gut flora is mainly known for its effect on digestive function, it is now apparent that maintaining a healthy bacterial balance is incredibly important to immune function, mental health, and likely many other aspects of health that we have yet to discover.

The spotlight on gut flora in recent years is well-deserved. Modern societies have become over-sanitized, wiping out the good bacteria with the bad, and dietary sources of good bacteria have almost disappeared. This lack of adequate "friendly bacteria" has also been exacerbated by factors like antibiotic treatment, birth control pills, radiation therapy, constipation, and diets that disrupt intestinal ecology. Since our diet has a major influence on the profile of the intestinal flora, antagonists to friendly bacterial proliferation will result in an overgrowth of coliforms and other "unfriendly" bacteria. Friendly bacteria are responsible for defending your body against disease and infection. They keep bad bacteria in check, preventing overgrowth and infection. Healthy bacteria are also responsible for regulating overall immunity, with several studies showing associations between probiotic supplementation and reductions in illness.

Some of probiotic bacteria's most direct roles involve digestion and gut health. Intestinal flora is responsible for the overall health and integrity of the intestinal lining, including the proper absorption of nutrients, excretion of wastes, and even production of some vitamins.

Additionally, there has been increasing evidence in support of a "gut-brain connection", showing strong ties between the state of intestinal flora and mental health. Healthy gut flora is found to play an important role in preventing various types of mental illness and maintaining healthy mood and cognition.

Probiotic Supplementation

Probiotic supplementation is useful in restoring or maintaining bacterial balance, especially when fermented foods are not consumed regularly, or when they are not strong enough to address the issue at hand. There are several factors that may compromise the integrity of your gut bacteria. For example, when you consume processed foods, refined sugars, and alcohol or use pharmaceutical antibiotics, the natural ecosystem of the digestive tract is disrupted. This creates a state of *dysbiosis* in which good bacteria may be hindered and pathogenic strains may thrive. Antibiotics are especially destructive to gut health. While sometimes necessary, and even life-saving, it's extremely important to limit their use, as antibiotics destroy (almost) all bacteria, good and bad, in their path. This creates not only large-scale issues such as antibiotic resistance, but also has an extremely negative impact on each individual's overall health. Upon killing beneficial bacteria, digestive processes are often in disarray, the immune system becomes weakened, and you are more susceptible to diseases and infections until your body rebuilds its natural defenses. The solution is to restore the good bacteria levels in your gut, as gently and as soon as possible.

Most healthy individuals are encouraged to periodically take a high quality multi-strain probiotic supplement in order to keep gut ecology strong. In cases of illness or serious digestive disorders, probiotic supplementation can be extremely beneficial, although it is best to work with a practitioner who is able to recommend the most suitable probiotic strains in combination with an appropriate diet and supplement regime.

At the very least, one should supplement with a probiotic formula during and/or after taking antibiotics. We suggest supplementing with a probiotic upon starting a course of antibiotics, and for at least 30 days after the prescription is finished. Probiotics are best taken a half hour before meals, and at least two hours apart from any antibiotics. Instructions may vary depending on the type of supplement. If gas or bloating is experienced, it likely indicates that your digestive system is adjusting to the change. Any minor side effects should clear up quickly, usually within 10 days.

Fermented Foods

Fermentation is a valuable tool that has been used for thousands of years, mainly for the purposes of food preservation, alcohol production and culinary innovation. Today, fermenting foods remains an excellent way to preserve crops for consumption year round. Interestingly, these products of ancient food preservation techniques are also found to have some profound health benefits, and are quickly re-gaining popularity as functional foods to enhance human health.

The process of fermentation involves the consumption of sugars by microorganisms like bacteria or yeast, resulting in the production of lactate, ethanol, carbon dioxide, and other metabolites. This can be achieved naturally or through the use of a culture starter. Depending on the types of foods, different bacterial and yeast cultures may be used, resulting in varying tastes and health benefits. There is also a wide variety of foods that are commonly fermented, and many of them have long histories of traditional use in certain cultures. Common ones include cultured dairy products, vegetables, grains, soy and tea (see Figure 1). Many of these products are found at restaurants, grocery stores and health food stores, but they are often very easily made at home as well. When buying any pre-made fermented foods, ensure that you are choosing raw, unpasteurized forms that have retained their live bacterial cultures – otherwise known as the "mother".

The consumption of fermented foods, and the resulting beneficial bacteria, has been shown to have remarkable effects on overall health, including digestive function, immune function, weight management, mental health, nutrient synthesis and the prevention and treatment of several diseases. Research has uncovered some possible mechanisms of action, including the modulation of gut pH, competition with harmful bacteria, production of antimicrobial compounds and stimulation of immunomodulatory cells.

The addition of beneficial bacteria and yeast cultures may also improve the digestibility of foods by breaking down anti-nutrients, increasing bioavailability of some nutrients, and even reducing glycemic load by pre-digesting sugars. For instance, some foods that often result in digestive difficulty, like gas and bloating, may be much easier to digest and assimilate when fermented, as in the case of sourdough versus other breads.

Consuming fermented foods is an excellent way to boost nutrient absorption and improve overall health. Whether you're preserving foods in the off-season, dealing with a digestive disorder or just aiming to eat well for disease prevention, the incorporation of fermented foods can allow you to take one step closer toward optimal nutrition.

Figure 1: Common Fermented Foods, Main Ingredients and Estimated Geographic Location of Origin or Popularity[1]

Fermented Food	Main Ingredients	Geographic Location
Apple Cider Vinegar	Apples, apple cider	Unknown
Cortido	Cabbage, onions, carrots	El Salvador
Cheddar and stilton cheeses	*Penicilliumroqueforti, Yarrowialipolytica, Debaryomyceshansenii, Trichosporonovoides*	United Kingdom
Crème fraîche	Soured dessert cream *L. cremoris,L. lactis*	France

Dosa	Fermented rice batter and lentils *L. plantarum*	India
Fermented sausage	Lactobacillus, Pediococcus, or Micrococcus	Greece, Italy
Igunaq	Fermented Walrus	Canada
Kefir	Milk, kefir grains *Saccharomyces cerevisiae* and *L. plantarum*	Russia
Kimchi	Cabbage *Leuconostocmesenteroides*	South Korea
Kombucha	Black, green, white, pekoe, oolong, or darjeeling tea, water, sugar *Gluconacetobacter* and *Zygosaccharomyces*	Russia, China
Miso	Soybeans *Aspergillusoryzae*, Zygosaccharomyces, *Pediococcus*sp.	Japan
Pulque	Agave plant sap *Zymomonasmobilis*	Mexico
Sauerkraut	Green cabbage *L. plantarum*	Germany
Sourdough	Flour, water *L. reuteri, Saccharomyces cerevisiae*	Egypt
Surströmming	Fermented herring, brine *Haloanaerobiumpraevalens*, *Haloanaerobiumalcaliphilum*	Sweden
Wine	Various organisms, commonly grapes. *Saccharomyces cerevisiae*	Many locations dating back to prehistoric period

| Yogurt | Milk
L. bulgaricus, S. thermophilus | Greece, Turkey |

9

Micronutrients, Phytochemicals & Superfoods

"Adequate consumption of micronutrients – vitamins, minerals and many other phytochemicals – without excessive caloric intake, is the key to achieving excellent health." – Dr. Joel Fuhrman

It's no secret that consuming a nutrient-dense diet is important to health – but which nutrients should we be looking for? One of the most crucial factors in achieving a truly nutritious diet is variety. This means looking deeper than fats, carbohydrates and proteins and aiming for an array of different **micronutrients** and **phytochemicals**. These include thousands of compounds in foods that have been identified based on their various roles in human health. As naturally-occurring components of plants and animals, micronutrients and phytochemicals are proven to be most effective when consumed in those forms. Each type of food that we eat has a unique blend of these health-promoting components, with some foods containing much more than others.

In order to ensure adequate consumption of vitamins, minerals and phytochemicals, it's also important that the foods we eat are fresh, unrefined, and grown in healthy, rich soil. However, our foods are often lacking nutrient density due to modern issues like mass production, nutrient-depleted soil, long-distance importing, refining and processing. Considering growing rates of disease and decreases in nutrient consumption, it is now more important than ever to be mindful of our diets and the vitamins, minerals and phytochemicals that may (or may not) be in them.

Micronutrients

The term, "micronutrient" describes a class of substances, including vitamins and minerals, that are essential in trace amounts for normal growth, development and function. Compared with macronutrients – fats, carbohydrates and proteins – micronutrients are required in smaller amounts, with much greater variety, and have very different physiological roles.

Vitamins do not directly provide physical structure or caloric energy. Instead, these substances help to perform several other biochemical functions, such as facilitating metabolism, acting as coenzymes and creating energy from macronutrients. Most cannot be manufactured in the body, and therefore, must be present in the diet. Thankfully, vitamins can be found in several different plant and animal food sources.

Vitamins are categorized as either water-soluble or fat-soluble. *Water-soluble* vitamins mainly consist of Vitamin C and B vitamins, including: thiamine, riboflavin, niacin, pantothenic acid, pyridoxine, biotin, folic acid, and cobalamin. These nutrients are easily lost and excreted, and need to be consumed regularly in order to ensure sufficient amounts in the body. Due to their water-soluble nature, they are excreted when consumed in excess, and are therefore considered to have low potential for toxicity. Vitamins A,D,E and K are *fat-soluble*, meaning that they are best absorbed along with fats and oils. These vitamins are normally stored for future use, and may accumulate at toxic levels if continually consumed or supplemented in excess.

Minerals are considered the basic constituents of all matter, meaning that they cannot be reduced or broken down to simpler substances. In various combinations, they are consistent throughout animals, plants, earth and space. Minerals are used in a multitude of functions in the human body, some of which involve the structure of bones and various types of tissue. There are certain minerals, such as calcium and phosphorus that are present in the body in higher amounts, and are found mainly in the bones. Others, like sodium and potassium, are extremely important in trace amounts for functions like fluid balance and nerve conduction. Most minerals also have key physiological roles in metabolism, energy production, cell communication, immunity, muscle function and pH balance.

There are approximately 17 different minerals considered to be essential to human health, and several more that are beneficial in small amounts. Some minerals are more likely to be deficient than others. For example, magnesium, iron and zinc are often supplemented to ensure healthy nervous system function, oxygen transport, muscle function, immunity and fertility. Large spectrums of trace minerals can also be crucial for increasing alkalinity and maintaining overall health.

Phytochemicals

This class of nutrients refers to the health-promoting, biologically active compounds (aside from vitamins and minerals) that are found in plants. Plants are known to produce various phytochemicals to protect themselves, but it is now understood that humans can benefit from them in a similar way to protect their cells and organ systems. This encompasses a seemingly infinite list of compounds found in all sorts of fruits and vegetables, thousands of which have been discovered so far.

Many phytochemicals have been studied in detail and are proven to have significant effects on human health, with specific disease-preventing functions. These phytochemicals include major classes such as anticancer compounds, antioxidants, detoxifying agents, neuropharmacological agents and immune-potentiating agents. Several studies have even demonstrated roles of various phytochemicals in the prevention of specific diseases, such as heart disease, cancer and diabetes. Several antioxidants have also been studied in depth for their roles in cell protection, free-radical scavenging and longevity, protecting the body from damage due to aging, pollution, stress and physical exertion.

Phytochemicals are present in different amounts and proportions in each plant species. Concentrations will also vary among different parts of each plant. Depending on the type of chemical, levels may be higher in the roots, leaves, fruit, skin or seeds of a given plant. For this reason, it is useful to consume several different edible parts of a fruit or vegetable. For example, consuming apples along with the skin is crucial in order to obtain maximum nutritional benefit, including fibre that modulates digestion and sugar absorption from the rest of the fruit. Similarly, oranges and bell peppers are best consumed with the white, fibrous parts inside that are rich in bioflavonoids, working synergistically with vitamin C from the rest of the fruit.

Phytochemicals are also classified based on their chemical composition and function within the plant. Some of these chemical classes include alkaloids, flavonoids, phenolics, tannins, glycosides, terpenoids and saponins. Certain types are known to affect specific sensory aspects of a plant, and each class of compounds may consist of hundreds of different phytochemicals that are responsible for various colours, tastes and smells. This is why incorporating a wide range of foods with diverse colours and flavors will result in a broader intake of phytochemicals with varying health benefits.

The consumption of isolated, individual phytochemicals is well-researched; however, the general consensus is that phytochemicals in supplement form do not provide the same effects as those in dietary form. This is likely due to the synergistic effect of plant nutrients within their original systems. Therefore, the best way to ensure maximum nutrient density and disease prevention is to consume a wide range of whole plant foods on an ongoing basis. Nevertheless, individual phytochemicals and extracts have been found to have distinct biological activities, and are often effectively used to improve certain aspects of health, especially in cases of illness or imbalance.

Below are some examples of well-known phytochemicals that are especially beneficial to health.

Alpha Lipoid Acid is a powerful antioxidant that protects the brain, nervous system and eyes from free radical damage. It is often used to promote healthy blood sugar levels and prevent diabetic nerve damage. Additionally, it has been found to protect the mitochondria of cells, support energy production, decrease the effects of aging and enhance the utilization of other antioxidants.

Beta-1, 3 Glucan comes from the cell walls of baker's yeast. It fortifies and activates macrophages – some key players in the immune system. Macrophages hungrily attack bacteria, cancer cells, fungi and viruses that invade the body, and make us ill. Beta-1, 3 gluten also protects against free radical damage from radiation, like X-rays and UV rays. As such, it is a powerful antioxidant and immune modulator. More specifically, it aids in the reduction and prevention of radiation damage, lowers high blood cholesterol and triglyceride levels, and is used in complementary medicine treatments for chronic conditions, such as herpes, *Candida albicans*, Epstein-Barr Virus and HIV.

Carotenoids are a family of substances that give fruits and vegetable their natural colours. Alpha carotene, like its family member beta carotene, is converted to Vitamin A. Carotenoids protect plants and humans against environmental carcinogens, such as UV radiation, with powerful anti-cancer and antioxidant properties. *In vivo* studies have shown its ability to significantly reduce the number of cancerous tumors in animals. Alpha carotene appears to be more powerful than beta carotene in the protection it offers against free radical damage to eyes, liver, skin and lung tissues.

Co Q 10 or ubiquinone, is a powerful antioxidant extracted from Japanese cabbage. With a critical role in energy production at the basic cellular level, Co Q 10 helps to deliver energy and oxygen to cells. It is often recommended for the treatment of cardiovascular disease, angina, high blood pressure, hypertension, infections, irregular heartbeats (arrhythmia), athletic performance, mitral valve prolapse, and periodontal disease.

Curcumin is a powerful antioxidant and anti-inflammatory compound that is found in turmeric root. As one of the most potent plant anti-inflammatories, it is especially effective against joint pain, without the potential side effects of pharmaceutical non-steroidal anti-inflammatories (NSAIDs). In addition, curcumin appears to reduce cancer cell activity, and may be helpful as part of a treatment program for breast, colon and skin cancers. It also offers protection against free radical damage, has the ability to lower high blood cholesterol levels, and can reduce the risk of blood clots.

Hesperidin is a bioflavonoid, immune system builder and powerful antihistamine. It is mainly helpful in relieving symptoms of environmental allergies and supporting cardiovascular health. It is especially effective for the prevention of bruising, varicose veins and other circulation problems.

Lycopene is another powerful antioxidant and member of the carotenoid family, responsible for the red colour of tomatoes. It's often used for its ability to aid in the protection of the prostate gland; and is also associated with the prevention of cancers, including breast, lung and pancreatic cancer.

Quercetin is a bioflavonoid found in green tea, apples, red grapes, cranberries, citrus fruits and green leafy vegetables. It's a strong antihistamine, powerful antioxidant and natural anti-inflammatory. Studies indicate that it also has powerful anti-cancer properties, in addition to improving circulation and strengthening capillaries.

Resveratrol is an antioxidant found in grapes. It offers antifungal properties, reduces the rate of blood clot formation, prevents plaque formation in arteries and may be anti-carcinogenic, helping malignant cells to be restored back to their normal state.

Rutin is a bioflavonoid usually derived from eucalyptus. It is a member of the C-complex family, working synergistically with Vitamin C and other bioflavonoids, such as hesperidin and quercetin. It has anti-inflammatory, antihistamine, antiviral, anticancer and antimicrobial properties. It also aids in the maintenance of collagen, which is critical for supporting the outer layer of skin, and facilitates wound healing. Like hesperidin, it strengthens the capillaries and may be helpful in treating varicose veins, bruises and hemorrhoids.

Superfoods: incorporating micronutrients and phytochemicals into your diet

"Superfood" is a term that has come up often in recent years as a way to describe trendy (and seemingly miraculous) additions to one's diet. First, let's be clear about the true definition of a superfood and what that means for nutritional wellness.

A *superfood* is generally defined as any natural food that carries an exceptionally high nutritional value and is therefore particularly beneficial for health. This is sometimes synonymous with the terms, *functional foods* or *nutraceuticals*, which describe foods that can have medicinal benefits as a result of their health-supporting components.

However, it's important to keep in mind that no one food alone is sufficient for overall health or capable of curing illnesses on its own. Each food has a unique combination of nutrients in various amounts, and variety is of the utmost importance for health. There are thousands of foods available that contain varying levels of nutrients. Nevertheless, some foods are especially nutritious additions to a diet, as they contain very high amounts or broad spectrums of nutrients and phytochemicals that are known to improve many aspects of health. Choosing superfoods is a matter of nutritional efficiency. Consuming nutrient-dense foods that contain large amounts of nutrients per serving will improve your 'nutrient to calorie' ratio, leading to a state of optimal nutrition.

With so many different food choices available from all parts of the world, it can be difficult to identify the ones that are especially nutritious, and what they can do for our health. The idea behind the identification of superfoods or functional foods is to shine a spotlight on the food choices that can have a particularly strong effect on our health. Below is a list of a few of the most powerful and easily accessible. You are encouraged to try a large variety of whichever ones are suitable to your needs and your tastes, and incorporate them often.

Apple Cider Vinegar is produced using fermentation, preferably from organically grown apples. The sediment contains trace minerals like potassium, pectin, healthy bacteria and enzymes. It's important to use an unfiltered and unpasteurized apple cider vinegar, containing the "mother" in order to obtain all of these beneficial components. Apple cider vinegar is often used to enhance digestion by stimulating stomach acid and enzyme production, as well as inhibiting the growth of bad bacteria in the digestive tract.

Artichoke concentrate (cynarin) is known to protect and support the liver, much like its botanical cousin, milk thistle. It helps to reduce the risk of cardiovascular disease and increases bile production, which aids in the metabolism of fats.

Bee Pollen is a source of several life-supporting nutrients including amino acids, enzymes, vitamins and minerals. As a result, it supports energy production, helps to build resistance to diseases, enhances digestive function and facilitates optimal hormonal balance.

Bee Propolis is the sticky material that bees gather from trees to seal their hives with. It protects bees in the hive from infection and intruders, and may help to do the same for human health. Bee propolis is a source of bioflavonoids, vitamins, minerals, resins and other substances, and is beneficial for gum disease, mouth ulcers, sore throats and initial stages of a cold. It's also effective against herpes virus when applied to lesions, relieves pain and aids in wound healing.

CamuCamu Berry, an Amazonian fruit, is one of the best known whole food sources of Vitamin C, providing 2.4 to 3.0g per 100g of pulp. It is also a source of a range of bioflavonoids and antioxidants, including polyphenols and anthocyanins. Camucamu's high antioxidant capacity has been confirmed throughout several studies, showing promising applications for disease prevention and longevity. It is available in North America mainly in the form of powders as a great addition to drinks and smoothies.

Chia Seeds are a fantastic source of omega-3 fatty acids, protein, soluble fibre and antioxidants. Their high soluble fibre content makes them a valuable asset to digestion and detoxification. Due to their nutrient content and its gel-like consistency when soaked, one tablespoon of chia seeds acts as a great egg substitute in recipes. They can also be used to make puddings or added as a topping to almost any meal, drink or smoothie.

Chlorella (Chorellapyrenoidosa) is a single-celled fresh water micro-algae plant that is loaded with powerful disease-fighting nutrients like chlorophyll, nucleic acids (RNA/DNA), plus 19 amino acids (including all of the essential ones), as well as 20 vitamins and minerals. Chlorella acts as an excellent detoxifier, anticancer food and tonic for the cardiovascular system. It has also been found to raise protein albumin levels in the blood. Albumin is a powerful antioxidant and principal transportation system for minerals, vitamins, hormones, fatty acids, and vital nutrients in the body, as well as the "garbage collector" of toxins. It helps to transports toxic substances to the liver for removal from the body.

Cordyceps is a medicinal mushroom known for its effects on immune modulation, hormonal balance, stress-response regulation and energy enhancement. It contains a wide range of nutrients including B vitamins, polysaccharides, sterols, proteins and trace minerals. Various types of extracts are used for medicinal purposes, such as enhanced stamina and athletic performance, fertility and immune support.

Flaxseed is a rich source of ligans, fibre, alpha-linolenic acid (ALA), oleic acid, linoleic acid and other essential omega-3 fatty acids. It's beneficial for digestive and urinary disorders, lowers cholesterol and blood triglycerides, and helps in clot formation prevention. It also decreases homocysteine levels in the blood, which is thought to reduce the risk of heart disease. Due to its influence on hormonal balance, it also helps to reduce the effects of premenstrual syndrome and alleviate menopausal symptoms of vaginal dryness and hot flashes.

Green Tea is a pleasing beverage rich in antioxidants and polyphenols, which have potentially powerful anti-cancer and anti-oxidant properties. Green tea helps to stimulate repair of skin damage, inhibits cancerous tumor formation and reduce the risk of esophageal, lung, stomach, pancreatic and colon cancer. It may also prevent heart disease, high blood pressure, high cholesterol, improve HDL cholesterol levels and stop abnormal blood clotting.

Hemp (seeds or oil) is an excellent source of essential fatty acids, many of which help to reduce inflammation and are needed for optimal health. Its potential benefits include pain relief, reduction of arthritic inflammation, anti-cancer applications, reduction of heart disease risk, neuro-protective effects and even anti-depressant potential.

Lion's Mane (Hericiumerinaceus) is a mushroom that is known for its profound effects on the nervous system. Containing a range of nutrients and bioactive substances, it has been traditionally used to enhance cognitive function, including learning, memory, focus and mood. It has even been shown to promote nerve growth factor secretion, contributing to the health, maintenance, regeneration and rejuvenation of the central and peripheral nervous system. As a result, it shows promising applications for the support and prevention of several neurodegenerative disorders, which include common diseases like Alzheimer's, Multiple Sclerosis, and various types of behavioural and cognitive dysfunction.

Maca is a root of Peruvian origin with several notable health benefits including hormonal balance, fertility, mental and physical energy enhancement, and mood stabilization. Available in powders, liquids and various types of extracts, it is most commonly used to increase energy, fight oxidative damage and address ailments like fatigue, depression and sexual dysfunction.

Maitake mushroom is another powerful "healer", traditionally used in Asian medicine. Japanese researchers started examining the science behind this ancient remedy, and found that it's mechanisms of action include the activation of the body's natural defenders against cancer and viral cells – the T-cells. Maitake is often used for its cancer fighting properties, as well for decreasing the extreme fatigue and nausea often caused by chemotherapy. Its immune system boosting and balancing properties translate to increased resistance to several diseases.

Reishi (Ganoderma Lucidum) is one of the most powerful and widely used medicinal mushrooms, used in both ancient and modern medicine. In studies using mice, reishi extracts have been associated with reduced growth of cancerous tumors. It is also a popular heart tonic, thought to oxygenate several organ systems and body parts. Reishi's immune modulating and antihistamine actions make it beneficial for immune support, including the control of allergy symptoms. It is also found to help lower elevated cholesterol levels, prevent blood clots and even greatly lessen the symptoms of altitude sickness.

Royal Jelly is the milky white secretion of a specialized group of nursing bees during the first twelve days of life. It contains all the B vitamins, Vitamin A, C, D, E, minerals, hormones, essential amino acids, antibacterial and antibiotic elements. As a result, it is known for anti-aging and beauty enhancing properties. Royal jelly can also help to strengthen adrenal function, which is critical for mood, appetite, metabolism and sex drive. It has been used to improve texture and quality of skin, reducing fine lines and wrinkle formation. Royal jelly may also be helpful for asthma, pancreatitis, insomnia, liver disease, kidney disease, stomach ulcers, bone fractures and immune system function.

Shiitake mushroom (Lentinusedodes), another medicinal mushroom, has traditionally been used to fight several illnesses including cancer as well as several types of infections, due to its beneficial effects on the immune system.

Spirulina is a protein-rich microalgae and a nutrient-dense powerhouse, with one of the highest concentrations of nutrients among almost all other plants. This impressive nutrient profile includes essential amino acids, iron, Vitamin B12, chlorophyll, gamma-linolenic acid (GLA), linoleic acid, arachidonic acid and nucleic acids RNA and DNA. Spirulina is often used to aid in detoxification, and is a great addition when fasting. It can also improve the absorption of minerals, support the immune system, and aid in blood sugar stability, appetite control and weight loss.

PART III

Accessories for Achieving Nutritional Wellbeing

"You are not only what you eat, but what you think, and combine on a physical, psychological, mental and spiritual level through eating well, exercising and enjoying life." - Dr. Elvis

10

Digestion:
From Food to Nourishment

The process of digestion, and the enzymes that facilitate it, are just as essential as food itself.

The human body is complex and mysterious. It's constantly working to keep us alive and well, although most people are unaware of its functions and how our day-to-day actions affect it. Even if we are mindful of the foods that we put into our mouths, we may be inadvertently reducing that food's potential as it travels through our digestive tracts. Therefore, understanding the process of digestion is another important step in achieving nutritional wellness. Awareness of our own body is an extremely valuable asset in making the best decisions for our health.

Optimal health depends on optimal digestive function. Without the ability to properly break down food and absorb nutrients, even the most nutritious diet cannot support overall wellness. As famously stated by Hippocrates: "All disease begins in the gut". In fact, it is likely that almost every illness and symptom can be traced back to, or connected with, some type of digestive dysfunction. Unfortunately, digestive imbalances are not uncommon.

Four out of 10 people visiting their doctors are there because of gastrointestinal complaints, including symptoms like heartburn, diarrhea, excess gas, constipation, nausea and food sensitivities. Yet, the most important signs that may take weeks, months or years to appear are diseases due to insufficient nutrient assimilation by the body. However, many people may not even be aware that they are experiencing digestive imbalance, mistaking mild symptoms and subtle signals from their bodies as "normal".

There are several factors that negatively affect digestion. Of course, diet plays a major role. Regular consumption of a diet that is high in processed foods and contains inadequate fibre usually result in a sluggish intestinal tract, which may subsequently contribute to several more severe disorders including colitis, diverticulitis, irritable bowel syndrome, Crohn's disease or colon cancer.

Lifestyle factors such as repeated stress and inactivity also play major roles in digestive function. Stress, whether physical or mental, shifts your nervous system into survival mode, neglecting less urgent functions like digestion, and inhibiting the action of your digestive organs. For this reason, several digestive symptoms and disorders, ranging from indigestion to IBS, are linked to stress and anxiety. Your digestive organs also require regular, gentle physical activity in order to function optimally and prevent issues like slow digestion or constipation.

From Food to Nourishment

Digestion is commonly known as a process that begins in the mouth. However, the digestive wheels often start turning before food even enters the mouth. Sight, smell, mindfulness and preparation are important activities in the timeline of digestion. These senses send signals to the brain, indicating that it's time to prepare the rest of the digestive organs for what's to come. This is where the term "mouth-watering" comes from: the production of saliva at the smell, sight or even the thought of great food.

Once food enters the mouth or **buccal cavity**, it makes contact with saliva that is produced to initiate digestion. Saliva contains a form of amylase (or ptyalin), which is an enzyme that begins the digestion of starch. Chewing is another incredibly important, and often neglected, action. It's responsible not only for breaking down food, but signaling the release of stomach acid and enzymes (Note: this is why chewing gum on an empty stomach can wreak havoc on digestion!). Many people chew their food only enough for it to be swallowed, but it should be thoroughly broken down to almost liquid form so that it is properly digested, absorbed and assimilated as it moves along. After food is sufficiently broken down in the mouth, it then enters the **esophagus**, which is made of smooth muscle. When the muscle constricts, it pushes the food toward the stomach. This type of constriction in the digestive system is called 'peristalsis' - a wavelike contraction that propels food on to the next step.

When food (bolus) reaches the **stomach**, it must first pass through a narrow entrance called the lower esophageal sphincter, which prevents stomach acid from ascending into the esophagus and causing 'heartburn'. This phenomenon is commonly experienced by those who eat quickly without thoroughly chewing, or do not have sufficient stomach acid, causing discomfort and reflux. Once the food passes the lower esophageal sphincter, food enters the stomach. At this time, enzymes are released to start breaking down the food. Enzymes, pepsin and lipase, combined with hydrochloric acid(HCl), begin the process of breaking proteins down into smaller fragments, known as amino acids. As food molecules like amino acids and fatty acids are first released from the bolus, another small valve, called the pyloric sphincter, opens on the bottom end of the stomach. The bolus, now a watery consistency, moves into the first part of the **small intestine** or "gut".

The first part of the gut is the **duodenum**, a tube shaped like the letter 'U' turned on its side. The duodenum receives this semi-liquid bolus, which becomes trapped in the bottom of the 'U.' The cystic duct enters the right side of the 'U.' This large duct carries bile from the gallbladder and digestive enzymes from the pancreas, into the food bolus. These compounds penetrate the bolus, cleaving macromolecules into smaller fragments.

Bile, a bitter greenish-brown fluid, is secreted by the liver as a vital player in fat digestion. Bile is produced between meals in small amounts and is stored in the gallbladder. It stores about 600 mL of bile – more than the liver can produce during a high-fat meal. During digestion, the presence of fat in the duodenum triggers the gallbladder to begin a series of contractions. The stored bile releases out into the lumen of the duodenum, where it begins to emulsify the fatty acids. For this reason, anyone who is missing a gallbladder is encouraged to consider a bile supplement in order to ensure proper fat digestion.

The **pancreas**, located behind and below the stomach, is both an endocrine and exocrine gland, meaning that it releases hormones for direct action in the bloodstream, in addition to releasing enzymes through ducts elsewhere in the digestive system. The pancreas is responsible for the production of hormones insulin and glucagon, as well as somatostatin. The pancreas produces about 1200 mL of fluid per day, which is mostly released during meals. It is delivered to the duodenum through the cystic duct, along with bile. During meals, hormones released from the duodenum signal the gall bladder to release bile and trigger the pancreas to secrete digestive enzymes in pancreatic juice.

Enzymes

Every cell in the body has a use for enzymes, which facilitate the millions of biochemical reactions happening every minute. Each enzyme has a particular job to do. Vitamins, minerals and oxygen all need enzymes to make them useful. Without enzymes, plants and animals would not be able to live.

Here, we will focus on digestive enzymes, which allow the breakdown and absorption of the nutrients that we consume. While they trigger change, the enzymes themselves do not change. They convert food into components of sugars, amino acids, fats, starches, vitamins, minerals and numerous other nutrients including plant phytochemicals. They are the guides that direct each nutrient toward the correct tissues and cells. Each enzyme is needed for a very specific function. Also note that enzymes of one type cannot be substituted for or converted to another type. Therefore, the absence or shortage of a single enzyme can cause someone to go from a state of health to one of disease or illness.

Enzymes are categorized according to their purpose in the body. With digestive enzymes, they are known as the hydrolase group. Each enzyme acts on a specific food component, and is named based on what it acts on, simply by adding "ase" after the substance.

The four basic digestive enzyme types are:

1. *Amylolytic* or amylase: found in the intestines, pancreas and saliva; breaks down carbohydrates
2. *Cellulase*: breaks down cellulose (plant fibres)
3. *Lipolytic* or lipase: breaks down fats
4. *Proteolytic* or protease: found in the stomach, intestines and pancreas; breaks down proteins.

The following chart provides a quick view of some common food components and their corresponding enzymes.

Food Components	Enzymes that break them down
Proteins	Protease
Lipids (fat)	Lipase
Carbohydrates	Amylase
Starches	Amyloglucosidase
Maltose	Maltase
Sucrose	Sucrase
Lactose (milk sugar)	Lactase

Carbohydrates are broken down into smaller glucose molecules.
Proteins are broken down into amino acids.
Fats are broken down into fatty acids and glycerol.

Starch digesting amylase enzymes:

1. *Alpha-amylase* and *beta-amylase* process starches into sugars. Alpha-amylase is present in the saliva and pancreas, while beta-amylase is found in unprocessed raw vegetables and grains.
2. *Glucoamylase* and *amylase* process starches in the small intestines. They can digest thousands of times their own weight in starches.

Protein digesting protease enzymes:

1. *Bromelain*: naturally found in pineapple
2. *Pancreatin*: comes from animal pancreas, which works best in the small intestines
3. *Pepsin:* animal enzymes that break down proteins into amino acids
4. *Prolase*: from the papain in papaya
5. *Protease:* papaya
6. *Renin:* converts casein, the milk protein, into a usable form for the body and helps release the calcium, potassium, phosphorous, iron and other minerals found in milk
7. *Chymotrypsin* and *trypsin* (produced in the pancreas; aid in breaking down proteins)

Many enzymes are obtained through the consumption of fresh, live fruits and vegetables. Some especially excellent food sources for enzymes include: the aspergillus plant, avocados, bananas, papaya (papain), pineapple (bromelain), mangoes and sprouts. Other great foods to improve digestive function include fermented foods like sauerkraut, kombucha or apple cider vinegar, which can increase stomach acid production, and contributes beneficial probiotic cultures.

If digestive function is hindered and enzymes are depleted, a digestive enzyme supplement may help for either occasional or regular use until digestion function is restored. A full spectrum enzyme supplement should contain enzymes that break down proteins, fats, carbohydrates, fibre and milk sugars. Below is a sample of a standard full spectrum digestive enzyme capsule, although there are several formulas available that may be more tailored to individual needs.

- Pancreatic protease (acid stable)
- Lipase
- Alpha amylase
- Amyloglucosidase
- Cellulase
- Hemicellulase
- Lactase

Pancreatic enzymes include chymotrypsin, trypsin, amylases, lipases, and nucleases. Chymotrypsin is a powerful enzyme that cuts small proteins into smaller, 20 to 60 amino acid fragments called polypeptides. Proteins are therefore broken down into amino acids. Trypsin has a very similar action. During the hours following a high-protein meal, these polypeptides are slowly reduced further in size until they consist of peptides: chains of two to 10 amino acids. After the duodenal phase of digestion, the nearly fully liquefied contents are propelled deeper into the intestine by peristalsis.

Intestinal Action

The intestinal system is responsible for several digestive functions, including break down of food components, assimilation into the bloodstream for distribution, and excretion of wastes. Therefore, maintaining a healthy intestinal system is extremely important to overall health. This should involve the maintenance of beneficial gut bacteria, the proper functioning of all other digestive tasks before this point, and of course the consumption of fresh, healthy, nutrient dense foods including plenty of fibre, water and oils.

The intestinal lining receives all of its nourishment via arteries that transpierce the intestine muscles. The bloodstream is responsible for nourishing and maintaining the health and functions of the glands that line the inner surface of the intestines.

Intestinal muscles surround and encircle the intestinal tube, produce the alternating contractions and expansion that push food and fecal matter through the length of the bowels. Peristalsis, the undulating flushing motion produced by the intestinal muscles, can become weak and sluggish, or sometimes may be over-stimulated, hypertensive and contracted, creating spasticity. Excessive contractions (spasms) of the muscles may unduly constrict the blood circulation. There are several factors that may interfere with peristalsis and overall intestinal function. This includes stress, nutrient deficiency, toxicity, food pathogens, poorly balanced gut bacteria and dehydration.

The intestinal system is a complex and intricate ecosystem, with a vast assortment of microorganisms living within it and contributing to its function. The gut consists of the largest amount of bacteria, and the greatest number of strains compared with any other area of the body. Therefore, this ecosystem requires balance in order to thrive and contribute to optimal digestion. If this balance is thrown off by factors like antibiotic use, poor diet, or impaired function of the upper digestive tract, pathogenic bacteria may overgrow, creating a vicious cycle as digestive function worsens. For this reason, maintaining healthy intestinal flora is likely one of the most important factors in achieving optimal digestion.

The Liver

With a long list of crucial tasks, the liver is an extremely important organ for not only digestion and metabolism, but also for several other physiological functions. The liver is responsible for filtering every single substance that we consume or come into contact with. It converts nutrients into optimal forms for use throughout the body, stores them for future needs or prepares them for excretion. It helps to regulate several aspects of metabolism and endocrine function, from energy storage to hormone production. The liver is also well known for its role in detoxification – helping to break down and remove unneeded or dangerous substances from the blood and safely eliminate them.

Detoxification is one of the liver's most notable roles. In modern societies, there has been a dramatic increase in exposure to toxic substances like synthetic chemicals, food additives, heavy metals and other pollutants. As a result, there has been an increased interest in stimulating detoxification through natural cleanses. While gentle "cleansing" may be helpful in certain instances, it is not recommended to use products to suddenly alter or stimulate detoxification processes without consulting a practitioner, especially in a state of poor health. Diet and lifestyle changes, along with some supporting foods and herbs, are normally more effective methods for optimizing detoxification and overall health in a safe and sustainable way.

Food and lifestyle recommendations for supporting liver health and detoxification

- Sulphur-rich vegetables like cabbage, Brussels sprouts, garlic and onions
- Herbs and spices: cilantro, dandelion root and leaf, nettle, burdock, milk thistle
- Soluble and insoluble fibre (ex. chia seeds)
- Gentle exercise to increase lymphatic flow and blood circulation (ex. yoga)
- Drink plenty of water, including warm water with fresh lemon
- Avoid alcohol, caffeine, processed foods and harsh synthetic chemicals found in cosmetics, etc.

Tips for Optimal Digestion

Foods
- A variety of fresh and/or raw fruits and vegetables, providing natural enzymes, fibre and micronutrients that aid in metabolism
- Fermented foods

- Sprouted foods (vegetables, seeds, grains)
- Fresh apples
- Pineapple
- Chia seeds
- Flax seeds (whole and ground)
- Jerusalem artichoke
- Apple cider vinegar
- Fresh lemon juice
- Ginger
- Cayenne pepper
- Herbal teas and warm liquids
- Unrefined plant oils, omega-3 fatty acids
- Psyllium husk

Lifestyle Adjustments

- Drink adequate water, warm or room temperature, and away from meals if possible to avoid dilution of stomach acid.
- Eliminate or reduce foods with refined sugars, preservatives, trans fats or other ingredients that may be difficult to digest, including irritants such as caffeine, alcohol, high amounts of dairy or any other known sensitivity.
- Drink one cup of warm water with fresh lemon juice in the morning, before eating.
- Incorporate vigorous exercise three to four times a week for 30 minutes.
- Reduce stress and calm the nervous system using natural modalities (i.e. massage, deep-breathing, yoga, tai-chi, qigong, counselling, laughter and hydrotherapy).
- Take time and care in preparing and enjoying meals.

Natural Supplements

- Probiotics: a multistrain formula including strains like *Lactobacillus acidophilus* and *Bifidobacterium longum*

- Digestive enzymes: lipase, amylase, lactase, sucrase, maltase and amyloglucasidase.
- Fibre: blend of soluble and insoluble psyllium husk powder, 500mg capsules three times a day with 8oz of water.
- Bromelain: 500mg two times daily with meals.
- Papaya: chewable one tablet with or immediately following each meal.

In some cases of digestive illness, upset or irritation:

1. Peppermint (unless experiencing reflux)
2. Ginger
3. L-glutamine
4. Marshmallow root
5. Slipper Elm
6. Pure aloe leaf (inner filet)
7. Deglycyrrhizinated licorice extract (DGL)
8. High quality or high potency probiotics (ex: 50 Billion + CFU)

11

The Art of Food Combining

In naturopathic medicine, the basis of food combining involves using principles of science and logic to enhance not only digestion, but most importantly, absorption of nutrients.

Many have utilized the practice of carefully combining foods in a particular way in order to relieve digestive issues, regain health, lose weight, increase energy levels, and keep the digestive tract more stable to prevent illness and disease. In addition to proper food combining, it is imperative to address other factors that can contribute to reduced digestive capabilities as well, such as overeating, eating when stressed, or eating before strenuous exercise. In addition, processed foods, excessive alcohol, coffee or tea can hinder proper digestion.

For many people, choosing the right foods can be difficult enough, and combining them in specific ways is not always feasible. However, food combining is an excellent complement to other diet and lifestyle techniques in order to achieve the most ideal and efficient digestive function possible. It can also be a key step in restoring a damaged digestive system or addressing specific illnesses. When practiced as often and as vigilantly as one's lifestyle will allow, the results can be fantastic.

When we eat foods such as meat, potatoes or fatty foods like vegetable oils, they must be broken down into smaller molecules before absorption into the blood can occur. Digestive enzymes cause a specific chemical change in food components, such as starches, proteins and sugars, whereby they convert them into substances the body can use to perform daily biochemical functions. Everything we eat needs enzymes to assist in digestion to convert meals into nutrients, vitamins and minerals.

Due to the fact that each food component is best digested and absorbed in particular conditions using specific enzymes, it is not always wise to combine several different types of foods at any given time. The goal of food combining is to give the most ideal digestive conditions for each food in order to make the process as smooth as possible, and get the most out of each nutrient.

9 General Rules for Proper Food Combining

1. Do not eat fruits with meals. For example, if you eat melons, eat them alone, as fruits are best eaten on an empty stomach. Ideally, they should be eaten 20 to 30 minutes before meals, as they take less time and energy to be thoroughly digested.

2. Do not eat sweet fruits or sub-sweet fruits with acidic citrus fruits. In general it is best to eat fruit alone since it digests quickly. Fruit does not digest when eaten with other foods in the stomach and cause putrefaction. Foods digest at different rates and ingesting an improper mix of foods can cause fermentation within the digestive system, slowing transit time; leading to bloating and possible bacterial imbalances. Acidic fruits like grapefruit are best to eat alone. However, they can be consumed with a sub-acid fruit like blueberries. Sub-acid fruits, such as sweet apples, apricots, cherries, mangoes, nectarines, pears, papayas and berries, can be mixed with either acid or sweet fruits.

3. Do not eat proteins with carbohydrates. The digestion of carbohydrates (starches and sugars), and of protein is very different. An alkaline pH is ideal to break down carbohydrates, whereas a lower, more acidic pH is ideal to break down protein into amino acids. Combining them can interfere with digestion, causing increasing acidity in the stomach. An acid process (gastric digestion) and an alkaline process (salivary digestion), cannot be carried on efficiently and simultaneously in the body. Thus, as the rising acidity of the stomach contents occur, it hinders carbohydrate digestion, resulting in fermentation.

4. Do not eat carbohydrates with acidic foods. Ptyalin is an enzyme which only acts in an alkaline medium. So if one consumes acid foods, ptyalin is destroyed by the mild acid. Therefore, acids not

only prevent carbohydrate digestion, but they also favour their fermentation and putrefaction.

5. Do not eat fats with proteins. When eating fats, the fatty acids decrease the activity of the gastric glands and gastric juices, and decreases pepsin and hydrochloric (HCL) acid. Therefore, it inhibits proper functions needed to digest meats, nuts, eggs or other protein.

6. Do not eat proteins with acid fruits. Acidic fruits reduce protein digestion because they inhibit the flow of gastric juice. However, acid fruits can be combined with high protein fats, such as avocado, cheese or nuts since these protein foods do not quickly decompose in this situation.

7. Do not eat when stressed or upset. One needs proper circulation and production of certain enzymes in the body to readily break down foods consumed, which is often inhibited in moments of stress. This can result in putrefaction, leaving food to ferment and increase toxins.

8. Do not overeat or consume sugar, jams, honey, syrups, cakes, cookies, pies, donuts or boxed cereals. Not only will they lead to inflammation, but will produce fermentation, along with an increased risk of developing Type 2 diabetes and obesity.

9. Do not eat quickly. Rather, try to spend quality time to eat in a relaxed atmosphere, and it is better to eat with others in social and family surroundings.

Food Combining Chart for Good Digestion

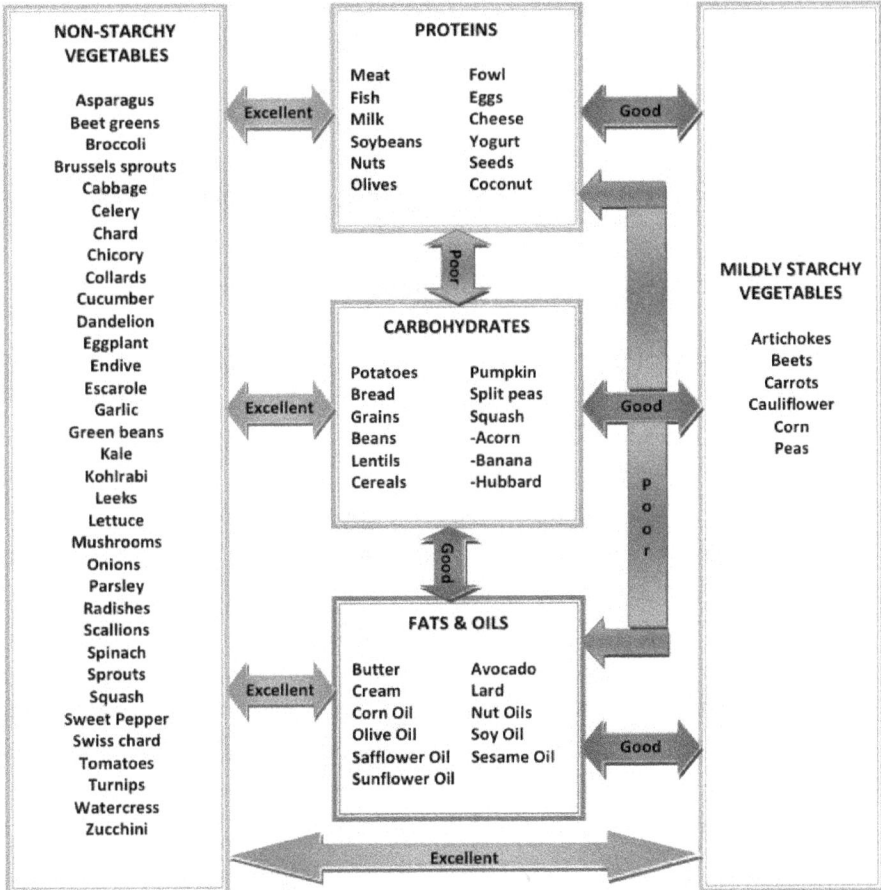

NON-STARCHY VEGETABLES

Asparagus
Beet greens
Broccoli
Brussels sprouts
Cabbage
Celery
Chard
Chicory
Collards
Cucumber
Dandelion
Eggplant
Endive
Escarole
Garlic
Green beans
Kale
Kohlrabi
Leeks
Lettuce
Mushrooms
Onions
Parsley
Radishes
Scallions
Spinach
Sprouts
Squash
Sweet Pepper
Swiss chard
Tomatoes
Turnips
Watercress
Zucchini

PROTEINS

Meat	Fowl
Fish	Eggs
Milk	Cheese
Soybeans	Yogurt
Nuts	Seeds
Olives	Coconut

CARBOHYDRATES

Potatoes	Pumpkin
Bread	Split peas
Grains	Squash
Beans	-Acorn
Lentils	-Banana
Cereals	-Hubbard

FATS & OILS

Butter	Avocado
Cream	Lard
Corn Oil	Nut Oils
Olive Oil	Soy Oil
Safflower Oil	Sesame Oil
Sunflower Oil	

MILDLY STARCHY VEGETABLES

Artichokes
Beets
Carrots
Cauliflower
Corn
Peas

Arrows: Non-Starchy Vegetables ↔ Proteins: **Excellent**; Proteins ↔ Mildly Starchy Vegetables: **Good**; Proteins ↔ Carbohydrates: **Poor**; Proteins ↔ Fats & Oils: **Good** (vertical) / **Poor**; Non-Starchy Vegetables ↔ Carbohydrates: **Excellent**; Carbohydrates ↔ Mildly Starchy Vegetables: **Good**; Carbohydrates ↔ Fats & Oils: **Good**; Non-Starchy Vegetables ↔ Fats & Oils: **Excellent**; Fats & Oils ↔ Mildly Starchy Vegetables: **Good**; bottom: **Excellent**; right vertical: **Poor**

Fruits are best when eaten separate from other foods on an empty stomach. It is best to eat melons and sweet fruits separately. Fruit makes an awesome breakfast and an energetic start to the day.

ACID FRUITS		SUB ACID FRUITS		SWEET FRUITS		MELONS
Lemon	Lime	Apples	Pears	Bananas	Raisins	Cantaloupe
Orange	Tangerines	Cherries	Nectarines	Grapes	Prunes	Honey dew
Raspberries	Pomegranate	Tart Grapes	Mangoes	Dried fruits	Figs	Watermelon
Pineapple	Grapefruit	Huckleberries	Sweet Plums	Dates		Casaba
Blackberries	Strawberries	Kiwi	Apricots			Musk
Kumquat	Sour Plums	Papaya	Fresh Figs			Persian
Sour apples		Peach				Crenshaw

12

Nutritional Supplementation

When and How To Choose Supplements

In cases of illness or imbalance, nutritional supplementation may be crucial for restoring balance and replenishing low reserves. However, it is important to keep in mind that all supplements are not created equally. The supplement market is becoming just as heavily saturated as the food market, with a very wide range of choices available. Most often, drastic price differences exist for a very good reason. Cheaper supplements are not necessarily better than none at all.

Close attention should be paid to sources, non-medicinal additives and fillers. For example, synthetic nutrientsare usually bound to other elements in order to be produced in the form of a supplement. Calcium carbonate, one of the cheapest and most common forms of calcium, is not only much less absorbablethan other forms, but can even create other health issues when deposited in other areas of the body. Certain fillers and additives may also be doing more harm than good by either hindering absorption or negatively impacting other aspects of health. Some supplements have even been shown to bypass digestion and absorption altogether, likely due to tough shellac coatings or capsules that cannot be properly broken down. For these reasons, it is important that you choose any necessary supplementation wisely, and speak with a trusted practitioner about the safest and most effective options available.

Research has shown that supplementation can be effective in some cases, although it is not nearly as effective as a well-rounded, nutritious diet. The reality is that most nutritional supplements are synthetically made, and while some forms may be safer and more effective than others, none of them can truly replace whole food nutrition. There are several differing professional and scientific opinions when it comes to synthetic supplementation, and the verdict seems to vary frequently. With so much left to learn about supplementation and human health, sticking to whole foods can be seen as a safer and more natural approach to wellbeing. Ideally, each nutrient should be consumed with the specific foods where it is found naturally, so that it accompanies the synergistic system in which it normally appears.

The use of superfoods can be an excellent way to address nutritional deficiencies without compromising safety or quality. This may include whole food concentrates or powders that are carefully dried or minimally handled for maximum nutrient preservation, using only natural, organic ingredients that are naturally high in certain nutrients. For example, foods like spirulina or moringa may be taken in a powder form as a source of a large spectrum of nutrients – acting as a natural multivitamin.

Supplementation can have an important role to play in overall health, especially for certain nutrients that many diets do not adequately address. Nutritional supplementation may also help to compensate for some of the nutrient depletion that affects our food supply. Nevertheless, it is clear that eating fresh, whole, nutrient-dense foods is by far the most important step to achieving overall nutritional wellness.

Important Dietary Components to Consider Supplementing

While most nutritional needs should be addressed by the foods found in a nutritious, well-rounded diet, there are some essential components that even healthy diets may be lacking, due to diminished nutritional value in our food supply, as well as increased nutrient demands and depletion. With such a vast array of supplements available, it is difficult to determine which ones are truly necessary.

Ideally, therapeutic supplement use should be tailored to individual needs. Working with a healthcare practitioner is the best way to create an effective and suitable diet and supplement regime, especially when illness is involved. Of course, moderation is key – more isn't always better. Caution should also be exercised when combining use with other supplements or medications. In general, it's best to consult with a practitioner to determine which nutrients you may be low in. However, there are a few specific nutrients that almost everyone should pay special attention to. Below are a few of the most common dietary components that may be missing from the average diet.

Omega-3 Essential Fatty Acids

As indicated by their name, essential fatty acids like omega-3 are crucial building blocks of human health that must be consumed from external sources, due to the fact that they are not produced in the body. With a long list of functions and health benefits, omega-3 fatty acids are likely one of the most important types of fatty acid for human health, and normally one of the hardest to obtain through the diet. Although there are plenty of healthy plant-based fats that can provide omega-3 fatty acids, the amount that the average person can effectively use from these sources are often quite low. Omega-6 fatty acids, on the other hand, are more abundant. The problem is that most people consume more than enough omega-6 fatty acids, and although these are also essential, a surplus can result in an imbalance that presents issues such as increased inflammation and compromised membrane health.Therefore, increased omega-3 intake is sometimes required to balance the ratio of omega-3 to omega-6.

For this reason, supplementing omega-3s in the form of fish oil, or a vegetarian source like algae oil, is an excellent way to improve overall health and prevent a wide variety of common health conditions. It's important to look for products that use clean and sustainable sources such as anchovies, sardines, cod liver or algae, and to ensure that the company has strong quality control policies, including third party testing to rule out oxidation, rancidity or contamination. Opting for an oil rather than a capsule helps to ensure a better price point and a higher dose per serving, as well as less additives and more optimal freshness in some cases. Some supplements will list milligrams of total fish oil, but be sure to look for labels that indicate amounts of EPA and DHA, especially for a therapeutic use like inflammation control. Ratios vary between products, but a higher EPA:DHA ratio is usually more desirable for inflammation control, whereas a higher DHA content is often recommended for nervous system or eye development, in cases like prenatal care.

Probiotics

As residents of virtually every surface of the human body, healthy bacteria plays a major role in all aspects of human health, including digestive function, immunity and mental health. Fermented foods can contribute some valuable bacterial cultures, although most of us are not consuming nearly enough of them. There are also several dietary, lifestyle and environmental factors that take a toll on gut flora and disrupt the balance of our digestive ecosystem. For this reason, most people can benefit from taking a probiotic supplement at one time or another, especially during or following antibiotic use. Supplements vary greatly in terms of the types of strains, strength (number of viable bacteria cells), sources and production methods. Certain strains may be more important for specific conditions, so it's a good idea to ask your healthcare practitioner or a health food store consultant about which probiotic supplement is best for you. Each strain will normally have an affinity to populate a certain area of the human body. For example, most supplements for general digestive health will typically contain some *Lactobacillus acidophilus* strains, as well as *Bifidobacteriumbifidum* strains, which are intended to act on the digestive tract, including the large intestine. Look for strengths that are listed in billions of colony forming units (CFUs). Most options range from millions up to hundreds of billions. Stronger probiotic supplements are usually recommended following digestive upset, antibiotic use, or other medication use that may affect gut flora. However, most mid-level strengths can be helpful additions at any time to improve digestive or immune function. For general health, supplementation may be recommended for 1 or 2 months of each year, and gut flora health can be maintained in between courses with a healthy diet including plenty of pre-biotic ("probiotic-feeding") fibres.

Vitamin D

Maintaining adequate levels of this nutrient is crucial to optimal health and has been shown to play a key role in mood regulation and disease prevention. Because Vitamin D is only synthesized in the skin in response to sunlight exposure, supplementation is often necessary, especially during the winter months. Vitamin D deficiency is alarmingly common among several populations, including those who live far from the equator and people who work overnight shift work. Most people in first world countries are deficient to some degree, due to a majority of hours spent indoors, as well as sun protection measures during time spent outside. Low levels of vitamin D are associated with an array of illnesses including seasonal depression, cancers, and many other physical and mental disorders. Vitamin D can be found in some mushrooms, as well as in the form of vitamin D3 (cholecalciferol). Most people will benefit from a dose of at least 1000IU, along with high quality fat or oil to enhance absorption and utilization.

Magnesium

As a mineral that is so vital for a multitude of functions in the human body, magnesium also happens to be one of the most commonly under-consumed nutrients. Some common symptoms of deficiency include: muscle cramps and muscle tension, headaches, migraines, constipation, anxiety, insomnia and cardiovascular issues. It is recommended to ensure adequate intake of magnesium-rich foods such as beans, nuts, leafy green vegetables, chlorophyll, blackstrap molasses and raw cacao. There are several types of synthetic magnesium supplements available and they can each behave very differently in the body. If higher amounts are needed and these needs are not being met by diet, a healthcare practitioner can help to determine which form may be best for you and your symptoms.

Vitamin C and B Vitamins

Stress is a frequent culprit when it comes to Vitamin C and B deficiency, quickly depleting stores that are needed for immune health, skin and tissue integrity, energy, metabolism and nervous system function. Vitamin C, as well as all of the B vitamins, are water soluble, and cannot be stored in the body for later use. Therefore, supplementation is often necessary, especially during periods of stress. When these nutrients are depleted, there can be serious implications for nervous system health, stress management, energy, hormonal health, mood and several other aspects of wellbeing. Some exceptional sources of Vitamin C include camucamu berries, amla berries and bell peppers. B vitamins can be found in an array of different foods as well, including several fresh fruits and vegetables, leafy greens, whole grains and algaes like spirulina.

Iron

Iron is another vital nutrient that plays an important role in circulation and energy. Deficiency can result in debilitating symptoms such as extreme fatigue. Supplementation can be important in cases of true deficiency, which is most common among women of childbearing age. However, iron can become toxic if taken in excess, and is not easily excreted. Therefore, it is best to consult a practitioner and have your levels tested before deciding to take an iron supplement. Food sources of iron include leafy green vegetables, nuts, seeds, dried fruits and animal products like red meats.

13

Nourishment Made Simple: Everyday Plant-Based Recipes

"Real Food doesn't have ingredients. Real food is ingredients"
– Jamie Oliver, Chef

Eating fresh, healthy food doesn't need to be complicated or time-consuming. In order to support a truly healthy life, it's important to find a balance. This means giving ourselves the nutrients we need to function optimally, but doing so in a way that is still convenient, sustainable and enjoyable. The following recipes present a few simple, fun and delicious ways to combine clean, nutrient-dense foods. You are encouraged to explore variations and make any necessary adjustments to suit you and your lifestyle. For example, you may occasionally want to swap in an animal-based protein or rearrange ingredients to follow food combining rules. These recipes, combined with the knowledge from previous chapters, can be used to cater to various taste preferences, dietary needs, sensitivities, budgets and seasonable availabilities.

Raw "Zoodle" Bowl

- 1-2 raw organic zucchinis, spiralized
- ¼ red cabbage, chopped
- ¼ avocado
- Shredded dried kelp
- ¾ cup non-GMO/organic tofu, lightly steamed
- 1 tbsp sunflower seeds
- 2 tbsp. tahini
- 3 tbsp coconut aminos
- 1 tbsp lemon juice

- 1 tbsp water

On top of fresh zucchini noodles*, add chopped cabbage and shredded seaweed. Tofu can be cut into small slices or cubes and quickly steamed in a pan at low heat along with 1 tablespoon of water.

In a separate bowl, combine 2 tablespoons of pure tahini or sesame seed paste, 3 tablespoons of coconut aminos* and 1 tablespoon of lemon juice. A pinch of Himalayan salt may be added as well, unless the coconut aminos have some added Himalayan salt or sea salt already. You can add 1-2 tablespoons of water to the mixture as well, depending on desired thickness.

On top of the noodles, cabbage and seaweed, add the steamed tofu, sliced avocado, sunflower seeds and tahini dressing as desired. (*Makes 1-2 servings*)

*Spiralizing zucchini and other raw vegetables is a quick and easy process that involves feeding the vegetable through a blade that cuts or shaves it into long "noodles", usually taking no longer than a minute. A simple spiralizer can be found at most stores that carry kitchen supplies for as little as $5, and is a valuable tool for making plant-based meals.

*Coconut aminos are a nutritious alternative to soy sauce, with a similar taste and an abundance of minerals, B vitamins, and amino acids.

Quinoa Harvest Salad

- 3 cups cooked tri-colour quinoa
- 3 small/medium local apples
- 1/3 cup raw pumpkin seeds
- 1/3 cup raw walnut pieces
- 1/3 cup unsweetened, dried cranberries
- sweet apple cider vinaigrette (see next recipe)

Combine cooked quinoa, raw nuts and seeds, cranberries and chopped apples in a bowl, and shake or mix thoroughly with approximately ½ cup sweet apple cider vinaigrette.
(*Makes 3-5 servings*)

Sweet Apple Cider Vinaigrette

- ¼ cup organic, unpasteurized, unfiltered apple cider vinegar (with the "mother")
- 1/3 cup hemp oil, flax oil, avocado oil or extra virgin olive oil
- 1 tbsp fresh lemon juice
- 1-2 tbsp raw unpasteurized honey
- Himalayan salt and fresh ground pepper to taste

Combine olive oil, lemon juice and apple cider vinegar in a blender for approximately 10 seconds, or shake to mix. Add 1-2 tablespoons of honey and blend again on high speed for at least 20 to 30 seconds or until combined and frothy. Lastly, add some Himalayan salt and fresh ground pepper to taste before shaking or blending once again. This mixture can be refrigerated in a jar or glass container for use with a variety of different meals.

****

Basic Buddha Bowl

- ½ cup wild or black rice
- 1 sweet potato
- 10-15 Brussels sprouts
- ½ cup sauerkraut or kimchi
- 2 cups spinach or kale
- 1 cup broccoli sprouts or other microgreens
- 2/3 cup chickpeas (canned or dry)
- 2 tbsp coconut oil
- 1 tsp turmeric powder, cayenne, or any other desired spices

After rinsing the rice, add 1-2 cups of water and bring to a boil, before letting simmer for 30 minutes or until finished (black rice or wild rice may take slightly longer to cook than white rice or brown rice). While the rice is cooking, wash the sweet potato and Brussels sprouts, and then slice before adding Himalayan salt (or any desired spices) to taste. Place them on a baking tray with a very light coating of coconut oil to avoid sticking and place in the oven for 12 minutes at 375 degrees F, flipping them over at six minutes.

Rinse the chickpeas (or cook, if using dried), and then steam* in a pan with a little bit of water, or ½ tsp of coconut oil and 1/4tsp of turmeric or other desired spices.

Spinach or kale may be lightly steamed with about 1 tbsp of water, in order to soften and inactivate any anti-nutrients (ex. goitrogens that may inhibit thyroid activity).

Add all ingredients on top of cooked rice, along with fresh broccoli sprouts or other microgreens. Sauerkraut (fermented cabbage) or kimchi can be added for an extra probiotic kick. These can be found pre-made at a grocery or health food store without artificial preservatives (bonus: make your own at home if possible!).

For some extra flavour, this bowl can be topped with a simple dressing of organic soy sauce/coconut aminos, or a splash of apple cider vinegar with a teaspoon of coconut oil.

The beauty of the Buddha Bowl is that you can easily swap the ingredients, using whatever fresh, colourful veggies you have in your fridge.

(Makes 2-4 servings)

*Chickpeas can also be roasted along with the sweet potato and Brussels sprouts, if you prefer them crunchy

****

Tropical Spirulina Smoothie

- 2 tsp spirulina powder
- 1 cup frozen mango
- ¼ avocado
- 2 cups coconut water

This one is super easy! Simply combine all ingredients in a blender. You may add more or less coconut water, depending on desired thickness. Frozen mangoes can be also be substituted with various other frozen fruits, such as bananas or local strawberries.

Baked Chickpea Quinoa Burgers

- 2 ½ cups chickpeas
- 1 ½ cup cooked quinoa
- 1 tbsp chickpea flour
- 1/2 red onion, diced
- 1/2 bunch black kale leaves, chopped
- 1/2 yellow bell pepper, diced
- 2 tbsp fresh lemon juice
- 1 tbsp water
- 2 tbsp coconut oil
- 1 tsp pink Himalayan salt
- 1 tsp fresh ground pepper
- 1 ½ tsp coriander powder
- 1 ½ tsp cumin powder

Blend soaked and drained chickpeas in a food processor until almost smooth. In a large bowl, combine blended chickpeas, cooked quinoa, and sautéed onions, pepper and kale along with the water, chickpea flower, and spices, mixing them together thoroughly.

Create small patties about the size of the palm of your hand. Carefully place each of them on an aluminum-free baking sheet with some coconut oil lightly spread on the tops and bottoms to avoid sticking. Bake for 10-12 minutes on each side at 425 degrees F, and let them cool before eating. These burgers are excellent on sprouted grain buns, on top of a salad, or even alone with a sauce like tahini.

****

Power Bites

- 5 Medjool dates
- 1 tsp raw cacao powder
- 1 tsp maca powder
- 2 tsp crushed raw walnuts or almonds
- 1 tsp cacao nibs
- 1 tsp chia seeds or hemp seeds

Using a food processor or blender, blend the dates first (using a bit of water if needed), in order to make a thick paste. Then add in the cacao and maca powder, followed by chopped walnuts, seeds and cacao nibs. When finished, use a teaspoon to measure small, bite-sized balls and roll, using the palms of your hands. Chia, hemp, cacao nibs and cacao powder can be rolled or sprinkled on after as well.

These bites can be served as a dessert or kept in the fridge for quick and energizing snacks throughout the week!

(Makes 5-10 servings)

REFERENCES

The Evolution of Nourishment

1. Pawlick, Thomas F. *The End of Food: How the Food Industry is Destroying our Food Supply – And What You Can Do About It.* Fort Lee, NJ: Barricade, 2006

2. Lima, G A, and et. al. *Calcium Intake: good for the bones but bad for the heart? An analysis of clinical studies.* ArchEndocrinolMetab., 2016, 60(3):252-63

3. Burton-Freeman, B.M. and H.D. Sesso. *Food versus Supplement: Comparing the Clinical Evidence of Tomato Intake and Lycopene Supplementation on Cardiovascular Risk Factors.* AdvNutr, 2014, 5:457-485

Grocery Shopping Tips

1. Pawlick, Thomas F. *The End of Food: How the Food Industry is Destroying our Food Supply – And What You Can Do About It.* Fort Lee, NJ: Barricade, 2006

2. Mercola, Joesph. *Artificial Sweeteners: More Sour Than You Ever Imagined*

3. Environmental Working Group, www.ewg.org/

4. Curl, C.L. et al. *Estimating Pesticide Exposure from Dietary Intake and Organic Food Choices: The Multi-Ethnic Study of Atherosclerosis* (MESA). Environ Health Perspect; DOI:10.1289/ehp.1408197, 2015

5. The Canadian Food Inspection Agency, *Method of Production Claims,* Apr. 2016, www.inspection.gc.ca/food/labelling/food-labelling-for-industry/method-of-production-claims/eng/1389379565794/1389380926083?chap=2

Dietary Essentials for Optimal Health

1. Haas, EM. *Staying Healthy with Nutrition*. Ten Speed Press, 2006

2. Lessard-Rhead, B. *Nutritional Pathology*. CSNN Publishing, 2013

Fats

1. Ali, E., e al. *The All In One Guide to ADD and ADHD*. AGES Publications Inc., 2001

2. Hibbeln, Joseph R. "Healthy Intakes of n-3 and n-6 Fatty Acids: Estimations Considering Worldwide Diversity." *American Journal of Clinical Nutrition 83 (6, supplement): 1483S-1493S;* American Society for Nutrition, June 2006 *PMID 16841858*

3. Okuyama, Hirohmi, et al. "3 Fatty Acids Effectively Prevent Coronary Heart Disease and other Late-onset Diseases: The Excessive Linoleic Acid Syndrome." *World Review of Nutritional Dietetics 96 (Prevention of Coronary Heart Disease)*: June 2006, *83-103. Karger. Doi,2007, 10.1159/000097809*

4. Covington, MB. *Omega-3 Fatty Acids*. American Family Physician. 2004, 70(1): 133-140

5. *McKenney, James M.; Sica, Domenic Prescription omega-3 fatty acids for the treatment of hypertriglyceridemia. American Journal of Health-System Pharmacy, March 2007, 64 (6): 595–605.* PMID 17353568

6. Leaf A, Kang JX, Xiao Y, Billman GE. "Clinical Prevention of Sudden Cardiac Death" *by n-3*

7. "Docosahexaenoic acid (DHA)" *University of Maryland Medical Center,* Cited on May 14, 2016, http://www.umm.edu

8. Haag M. "Essential Fatty Acids and the Brain." *Canadian Journal of Psychiatry,* 2003,48(3):195-203

9. Morris MC, Evans DA, Bienias JL, Tangney CC, Bennett DA, Wilson RS, Aggarwal N, Schneider J. *Consumption of Fish and N-3 Fatty Acid and Risk of Incident Alzheimer Disease.* Archives of Neurology, 2003,60(7):940-946

10. "Polyunsaturated Fatty Acids and Mechanism of Prevention of Arrhythmias by n-3 Fish Oils." *Circulation,* 2003,107:2646-2652

11. Trivedi, Bijal, "The Good, The Fad, and the Unhealthy" *New Scientist,* Sept. 23, 2006, pp. 42–49

12. http://www.hcsc.gc.ca/dhpmps/prodnatur/applications/licen-prod/monograph/mono_fish_oil_huile_poisson-eng.php

13. Wilson, PW, et al, "Prediction of Coronary Heart Disease using Risk Factor Categories." *Circulation 97,* 1998: 1837-1847

14. "What is Heart Disease?" *Heart and Stroke Foundation.* Cited on May 14, 2016
http://www.heartandstroke.com/site/c.ikIQLcMWJtE/b.3682421/k.48B2/Heart_disease__What_is_heart_disease.htm?gclid=CjwKEAjwmdu5BRCg1O3atDY0AQSJACKPgRK5qYF48QOAJ2EJusqqbBDPZSyXVVOoxGdFDu3vgAmdxoC60nw_wcB

15. Colman, J. "Why our Arteries Become Cogged with Age." *Life Extension Magazine,* Oct 2005

16. Gordon DJ, Probstfield JL, et al. "High-density Lipoprotein Cholesterol and Cardiovascular Disease. Four Prospective American Studies." *Circulation79 (1),* 2005: 8-15. PMID 2642759

17. "Detection, Evaluation and Treatment of High Blood Cholesterol in Adults (Adult Treatment Panel III) Final Report" (PDF).

National Institutes of Health. National Heart, Lung and Blood Institute, Oct. 27, 2008

18. "The Changing Face of Heart Disease and Stroke in Canada" *Health Canada, 2000.* Cited on May 14, 2016, httlp://www.hcsc.gc.ca/hpb/lcdc/bcrdd/hdsc2000/pdf/card2ke.pdf.

19. "High Blood Cholesterol: What You Need to Know". *National Cholesterol Education Program.* Oct. 24, 2008

20. Hendriks, H.F.J. Westrate, J.A., van Vliet, T. Meijer, G.W. "Spreads Enriched with Three Different Levels of Vegetable Oil Sterols and the Degree of Cholesterol Lowring in Normocholesterolaemic and Mildly Hypercholesterolaemic Subjects." *European Journal of Clinical Nutrition,* 1999,53:319-327

21. Weststrate JA, Meijer GW. "Plant-sterol Enriched Margarines and Reduction of Plasma Total- and LDL- Cholesterol Concentrations in Normocholesterolaemic and Mildly Hypercholesterolaemic Subjects." *European Journal of Clinical Nutrition,* 1998, 52:334-43

22. Ling, W.H., and P.J.H. Jones, *"A Dietary Phytosterols: A Review of Metabolism, Benefits and Side Effects." Life Sciences, Vol. 57.* pp. 1995,195-206

23. Groff J, Gropper S. "Advanced Nutrition and Human Metabolism" *3rd Edition. Belmont (CA):* Wadsworth/Thomson Learning, 2000

24. Shils ME, Olson JA, Shike M, Ross AC, Editors. "Modern Nutrition in Health and Disease" *10th Edition. Philadelphia (PA):* Lippincott Williams and Wilkins, 2006

Fibre

1. Alfieri, M A, et al. *Fibre intake of normal weight, moderately obese and severely obese subjects.* Obesity Research, Nov. 1995, 3(6):541-7

2. Aller, R, et al. *Effect of soluble fibre intake in lipid and glucose levels in healthy subjects: a randomized clinical trial.* Diabetes Research and Clinical Practice, 2004, 65(1):7-11

3. Alonso-Coello, P. et al. *Fibre for the treatment of hemorrhoids complications: a systematic review and meta-analysis.* The American Journal of Gastroenterology, Jan. 2006, 101(1):181-8

4. Åman, P. *Cholesterol-lowering effects of barley dietary fibre in humans: scientific support for a generic health claim.* Scandinavian Journal of Food and Nutrition, 2006, 50(4):173-76

5. American Association of Cereal Chemists (AACC). *The Definition of Dietary Fibre.* Cereal Foods World, 2001, 46(3):112-26

6. Anderson, BM, Gibson RS and Sabry JH. *The iron and zinc status of long-term vegetarian women.* The American Journal of Clinical Nutrition, Jun. 1981, 34(6):1042-8

7. Anderson JW, Allgood LD, Lawrence A, Altringer LA, Jerdack GR, Hengehold DA, et al. *Cholesterol-lowering effects of psyllium intake adjunctive to diet therapy in men and women with hypercholesterolemia: meta-analysis of 8 controlled trials.* The American Journal of Clinical Nutrition, 2000a, 71(2):472-9

8. Anderson JW, Allgood LD, Turner J, Oeltgen PR, Daggy BP. *Effects of psyllium on glucose and serum lipid responses in men with Type 2 diabetes and hypercholesterolemia.* The American Journal of Clinical Nutrition, 1999, 70(4):466-73

9. Anderson JW, Baird P, Davis RH Jr, Ferreri S, Knudtson M, Koraym A, et al. *Health benefits of dietary fibre.* Nutrition Reviews, 2009, 67(4):188-205

10. Anderson JW, Davidson MH, Blonde L, Brown WV, Howard WJ, Ginsberg H, et al. *Long-term cholesterol-lowering effects of psyllium as an adjunct to diet therapy in the treatment of*

hypercholesterolemia. The American Journal of Clinical Nutrition, 2000b, 71(6):1433-8

11. Anderson JW, Ferguson SK, Karounos D, O'Malley L, Sieling B, Chen WJ. *Mineral and vitamin status on high-fibre diets: long-term studies of diabetic patients.* Diabetes Care, 1980, 3(1):38-40

12. Anderson JW, Zettwoch N, Feldman T, Tietyen-Clark J, Oeltgen P, Bishop CW. *Cholesterol-lowering effects of psyllium hydrophilic mucilloid for hypercholesterolemicmen.* Archives of Internal Medicine,1988,148(2):292-6

13. Andoh A, Tsujikawa T, Fujiyama Y. *Role of dietary fibre and short-chain fatty acids in the colon.* Current Pharmaceutical Design, 2003, 9(4):347-58

14. Anti M, Pignataro G, Armuzzi A, Valenti A, Iascone E, Marmo R, et al. *Water supplementation enhances the effect of high-fibre diet on stool frequency and laxative consumption in adult patients with functional constipation.* Hepatogastroenterology,1998, 45(21):727-32

15. Ali, Elvis et al. *The All In One Guide to Natural Remedies and Supplements.* Ages Publication Inc., 2000

16. Ehrlich, SD, NMD. *Fibre.* University of Maryland Medical Center (UMMC), April 4, 2016

17. Enker, Warren MD. *Bowel Function - Dietary Fibre.* Mount Sinai, April 4, 2016

18. *It's About Eating Right – Fibre.* Academy of Nutrition and Dietetics, April 4, 2016

19. Threapleton DE, Greenwood DC, Evans CE, Cleghorn CL, Nykjaer C, Woodhead C, Cade JE, Gale CP, Burley VJ.*Dietary fibre intake and risk of first stroke: a systematic review and meta-analysis,* May, 2013, 44(5):1360-8

Probiotics and Fermented Foods

1. Ahmed, M, et al. "Impact of consumption of different levels of Bifidobacteriumlactis HV019 on the intestinal microfl." *The Journal of Nutrition, Health and Aging*, 2007, 11, 26-31

2. Ali, Elvis et al. *Natural Remedies and Supplements* AGES Publications, 2000

3. Bested, A.C. et al. "Intestinal microbiota, probiotics and mental health: from Metchnikoff to modern advances: part III – convergence toward clinical trials." *Gut Pathog*, 2013, 5:4

4. Chilton, S N, et al. "Inclusion of Fermented Foods in Food Guides around the World. Nutrients." Jan. 2015, 7(1): 390–404

5. Gopal, P K, et al. "Effects of the consumption of Bifidobacteriumlactis HN019 (DR10™) and galacto-Oligosaccharides on the microflora of the gastrointestinal tract in human subjects." *Nutrition Research*, 2003, 23, 1313-1328

6. Parvez, S., et al. "Probiotics and their fermented food products are beneficial for health. " *Journal of Applied Microbiology.* Jun, 2006:100(6):1171-85

7. Jorgen, Schlundt. "Health and Nutritional Properties of Probiotics in Food including Powder Milk and Live Lactic Acid Bacteria." *Report of a joint FAO/WHO expert consultation on evaluation of health and nutritional properties of probiotics in food including powder mild with live lactic acid bacteria.* Oct. 22, 2012

8. Sender, R. et al. "Revised Estimates for the Number of Human and Bacteria Cells in the Body." *PLOS Biology.* Aug. 2016, 14(8)

Micronutrients, Phytochemicals and Superfoods

1. Justi, K.C. et al. "Nutritional composition and Vitamin C stability in stored camucamu (Myrciariadubia) pulp." *Arch LatinoamNutr.* Dec. 2000, 50(4):405-8

2. Langley, P.C. et al. "Antioxidant and Associated Capacities of CamuCamu (Myrciariadubia). A Systemic Review." *Journal of Alternative and Complementary Medicine.* 2015, 21(1):8-14

3. Saxena, M. et al. "Phytochemistry of Medicinal Plants." *Journal of Pharmacognosy and Phytochemistry.* 2013, 1 (6): 168-182

4. Stamets, P. MycoMedicinals: "An Informal Treatise on Mushrooms." *MycoMedia Productions.* 2002

5. Tuli, H S, et al. "Pharmacological and Therapeutic Potential of Cordyceps with special reference to Cordycepin." *3 Biotech*, 2014

6. Zenico, T. et al. "Subjective effects of Lepidiummeyenii (Maca) extract on well-being and sexual performances in patients with mild erectile dysfunction: a randomised, double-blind clinical trial." *Andrologia.* 2009, 41(2):95-9

Food Combining

1. "Healthline. Factors influencing digestion and absorption of nutrients." Cited on Feb. 26 2016, http://www.healthline.com/hlbook/nut-factors-influencing-digestion-and-absorption-of-nutrients

2. *Dorland's Medical Dictionary.* "Digestion" Cited on Feb. 22nd, 2016, http://www.mercksource.com/pp/us/cns/cns_search_results.jsp

3. *Medline Plus.* Enzyme Cited on Feb. 22, 2016, http://www.nlm.nih.gov/medlineplus/ency/article/002353.htm

4. Bixquert Jiménez M. "Treatment of irritable bowel syndrome with probiotics. An etiopathogenic approach at last?" Rev EspEnferm Dig. Aug. 2009, 101(8):553-64.

5. *Medline Plus.* "Irritable Bowel Syndrome" Cited on Feb. 22 2016, http://digestive.niddk.nih.gov/ddiseases/pubs/ibs/

6. Brenner DM, Chey WD. "Bifidobacteriuminfantis 35624: a novel probiotic for the treatment of irritable bowel syndrome". Rev GastroenterolDisord. Winter, 2009, 9(1):7-15

7. Dolin BJ. "Effects of a proprietary Bacillus coagulans preparation on symptoms of diarrhea-predominant irritable bowel syndrome." Methods Find ExpClinPharmacol. Dec. 31, 2009, (10):655-9

8. Whorwell. PJ, et al. "Efficacy of an encapsulated probiotic Bifidobacteriuminfantis 35624 in women with irritable bowel syndrome." Am J Gastroenterol. July, 2006,101(7):1581-90

9. *Medline Plus.* "Fibre"Cited on Feb. 23rd, 2016, http://www.nlm.nih.gov/medlineplus/ency/article/002470.htm

10. Jonn Matsen ND. *Eating Alive: Prevention Thru Good Digestion* Vision Press. Jan. 1, 1991

11. Harvey Diamond, Marilyn Diamond. *Fit for Life* Grand Central Life and Style Hatchette Book Group. Aug. 16, 2010

ABOUT THE AUTHORS

Jaime Camirand is a Registered Holistic Nutritionist, Health Consultant and University of Guelph graduate with specializations in Nutritional and Nutraceutical Sciences, as well as Marketing Management. In light of rising rates of chronic diseases among so many people, including some very close to her heart, she has developed a passion for preventative approaches to health. Following years of experience working in conventional pharmacies, her focus is on nutritional wellness, along with the use of other supporting lifestyle practices. Her goal is to educate and empower individuals to achieve a healthier relationship with food, a stronger understanding of holistic and integrative health, and an overall state of sustainable wellbeing.

****

Dr. Elvis Ali is highly respected for his work in Naturopathic Medicine. Dr. Elvis, as he is affectionately known, has been in private practice for over 30 years, specializing in Chinese and sports medicine and nutrition. He lectures internationally, serves on *Alive's* Editorial Advisory Board, Member of OAND, CAND and OBACM, written several books and appeared on radio and television shows.

Dr. Elvis' credentials are impressive: Bachelor of Science, majoring in Biology, Licensed Acupuncturist, Doctorate in Naturopathic Medicine; Mind/Body Medicine at Harvard Medical School, Diploma in Homeopathic Medicine. He is passionate about educating people on complementary health and wellness, and non-intrusive options.

www.ingramcontent.com/pod-product-compliance
Lightning Source LLC
Chambersburg PA
CBHW071136280326
41935CB00010B/1253